The Jossey-Bass/AHA Press Series translates the latest ideas on health care management into practical and actionable terms. Together, Jossey-Bass and the American Hospital Association offer these essential resources for the health care leaders of today.

Guide to Effective Staff Development in Health Care Organizations

Patrice L. Spath, Editor

Foreword by James B. Conway

Contents

Part Three: Training Solutions: Case Studies

Tables, Figures, and Exhibits

. . . .

Tables

Figures

Exhibits

Foreword

James B. Conway

I f you are a busy health care executive, congratulations on pick-
ing up this book. At a time when the workday couldn't be longer
and the work demands more complex, it is in your best interest to
read it all the way through. The need for training in our health
care institutions is expanding exponentially, yet the dollars to support such training are not. It is crucial that as executives responsible for the best use of funds, we get maximum value from our
training dollars, recognize and understand the enormous potential
from training and the cost savings that can result from it, and focus
our efforts for maximum effectiveness. Without question, training
can contribute significantly to organizational and personal success.
But that doesn't just happen. Creating and sustaining a learning
culture and the accompanying training activities requires organizational leadership.

This book is written for health care executives as a guide toward
action-oriented results. In planning its content, some key assumptions were made about executives and their needs. The authors have
assumed that a vibrant learning environment is essential for organizational success. They strongly believe that executive leadership
is essential to the learning organization and that learning and training are challenging, if not impossible, without it. They also understand that no matter how talented a leader may be, leading a

learning organization is not an innate skill. For leaders to be effective in that role, they must learn how to do it and where to focus.
Leaders themselves must be good students and good teachers.

We need to know where the future of health care is heading, and
a vision of a dynamic learning environment will help keep us on
course. The key components of my personal vision are as follows:

- Organizational leaders participate fully in training
  as students, teachers, and supporters.

- Everyone recognizes that training is essential, not
  discretionary.

- Leaders understand the need to provide up-to-date
  resources for training in the form of staff, space, time,
  and employee benefits.

- Teaching and training are competencies to be developed
  and rewarded in staff at every level in the organization.

- Staff receive the training they need to be successful in
  the organization, using its systems and initiatives. This
  training begins before program implementation and
  continues into the future.

- Training programs are fashioned to meet prioritized
  institutional, programmatic, and departmental goals
  and with the active participation of leaders and staff.

- Training outcomes are measurable, are measured, and
  are reviewed.

- Technology is used effectively to support learning and
  reassessment.

- Staff have the opportunity to seek out training opportunities in-house or externally to support continuing
  education as well as to maintain current competency.

- Everyone should be encouraged to take day-to-day experiences and translate them into organizational improvement solutions.

- Training programs should be expanding, not shrinking.

What are the outcomes if this vision is realized? Three are of enormous importance:

1. *High-quality patient care and continuous improvement.* Effective competency assessment, training intervention, and in-service and continuing education allow for the provision of care that is more standardized, reproducible, and measurable. Instead of hoping, wishing, or "ordering" staff to do things right, the focus is on enabling through dynamic training. In this environment, when staff experience difficulties or failures in day-to-day operations, they use the learning potential of these events as a resource for improvement. In my vision, it is impossible to have breakthrough performance improvement in the absence of a learning environment.

2. *Successful change management.* Our organizations are all going through massive change. If we are committed to making improvements, such as those suggested in studies like *Crossing the Quality Chasm* (Committee on Quality of Health Care in America, 2001), even more massive changes will be needed. These changes will require significant resources. Organizations that place a high priority on learning will find change dramatically more successful because the efforts will have positioned staff for success.

3. *Improved retention and recruitment.* People come to health care to be successful, to be part of the solution, to make a difference, and the vast majority want to continue on that path. They want to learn, grow, do things right for the people they serve, and remain well prepared for the work of each day as well as for the next move, the next success. Employees—we executives, too—are attracted to organizations that position us for success and are alienated by organizations that position us for failure. Staffing shortages now and in the foreseeable future will make recruitment and retention key areas

of focus. Fostering an effective learning environment is a big plus in being perceived as an employer of choice.

Reference

Committee on Quality of Health Care in America, Institute of Medicine. *Crossing the Quality Chasm: A New Health System for the 21st Century.* Washington, D.C.: National Academy Press, 2001.

Preface

· ·

Peter Drucker (1993, p. 193) writes that the "basic economic resource . . . is no longer capital, nor natural resources . . . nor labor. It is and will be knowledge." Staff education and training is an important and valuable asset in a health care organization. Workforce development activities enhance employees' skills and help achieve health service goals. Education and training is also a critical component of a successful staff hiring and retention strategy. Training can also benefit employees by improving their incomes, advancing their careers, and enabling them to grow as people.

To survive in the increasingly competitive markets, health care organizations need employees with highly developed skills. Today's job descriptions for health care workers call for multiskilled people who can adapt quickly to new technology and learn new ways of performing tasks. Every health care organization faces the challenge of hiring and retaining people who meet these job requirements. As work in health care becomes more complicated and as hierarchical structures give way to lateral organizations, all employees will need retraining and retooling. To ensure quality and consistency, many organizations will need to strengthen internal staff training and development programs. A health care organization cannot maximize resources without focusing on its most important asset: employees.

There appears to be a growing realization among health care organizations that staff education and training programs must be improved. Having struggled through downsizing and budget cuts over the past several years, senior leaders are now seeing the unfortunate results of not having given the staff training function adequate priority during these turbulent times. Human resource and staff education departments have been among the hardest hit by job cuts in health care facilities.

Correcting past mistakes is made more difficult and yet more important by today's demographic and employment market trends. The health care workforce is aging rapidly, and in the next five years, many of its members will be eligible for retirement. Exacerbating the problem is the tight labor market, which makes attracting new employees—especially those in direct patient care positions—hard to do. All these signs point to an emerging crisis in the health care workforce. There is a solution, however, and senior leaders in health care organization must be part of that solution. Aggressive recruiting and quality training will succeed only when leadership is committed to a learning environment. Part One of this book covers the elements of a learning organization and the role of leaders in creating and supporting such a climate. In Chapter One, Anthony DiBella describes the context for learning in health care organizations and suggests how educational priorities can be established. A model for integrating all facets of staff education and performance evaluation is presented by Kathleen Heery in Chapter Two. In Chapter Three, Diane Boynton and Donald Sibery discuss the poignant transformation of Central DuPage Health, in Winfield, Illinois, into a learning environment.

There are numerous books on the technical aspects of staff development in health care organizations. This one is different. It is designed to provide the health care executive with an overview of staff training and education strategies to help leaders make informed decisions about program priorities. To begin this instructive process, Part Two of the book is devoted to training issues. In Chapter Four, Connie Kuykendall and Sally Zuel summarize the significant training issues health care organizations face. Chapters Five through Eight present key challenges in greater detail, along with solutions: selection of training methods, adult learning strategies, measuring the value of training, and critical components of an effective training program.

Throughout the country, a number of health care organizations have already begun to tackle the dilemmas of staff education and training. In Part Three, four case studies are presented to illustrate some effective training initiatives in health care organizations. Each case study is prefaced with short statements that describe the presenting problems, solutions, and results from each organization. In Chapter Nine, Christina Dempsey details the nurse scrub training program at St. John's Regional Health Center in Springfield, Missouri. The Web-based coding training program at Catholic Healthcare West is described by Gloryanne Bryant and Claire Dixon-Lee in Chapter Ten. The comprehensive staff education and training program at William Beaumont Hospital in Royal Oak, Michigan, is presented by Alice Speers, Karen Zaglaniczny, and Christine Zambricki in Chapter Eleven. In Chapter Twelve, Rebecca Petersen details a unique training collaboration among hospitals in Northern California.

Health care organizations can't hope to achieve their strategic mission goals without paying attention to the people factor. There are no results without talented people to put them in place. To transform an organization into a learning environment and set the stage for an effective staff education program, senior leaders must establish a learning vision and objectives and position staff educators to be strategic partners in the process. The organization must study the gaps between employee knowledge and skills and current and future needs. A plan of action must be designed to close those gaps with recruitment, education, succession planning, restructuring, or other means. Training programs must be aligned with strategic business goals and constantly reassessed on the basis of successes, failures, and changing organizational needs.

While staff educators can assess people's learning needs and develop training programs, there are no guaranteed results without leadership support. For staff development to be effective, senior leaders must have the will to follow through with resources and personal involvement. Staff education and training initiatives must be part of each health care organization's broader strategic planning effort.

Reference

Drucker, P. *Post-Capitalist Society*. New York: HarperCollins, 1993.

November 2001   Patrice L. Spath
                                                     Forest Grove, Oregon

The Editor

PATRICE L. SPATH is a health information management professional with extensive experience in health care performance improvement activities. She is a partner in Brown-Spath & Associates (www.brownspath.com), a health care publishing and training company based in Forest Grove, Oregon. During the past twenty years, she has presented more than 350 educational programs on quality improvement, case management, medical error reduction, and outcomes management topics.

Spath has written or edited more than 150 books and journal articles for American Hospital Publishing/Jossey-Bass Publishers, the National Association for Healthcare Quality (NAHQ), the American Health Information Management Association (AHIMA), Aspen Publications, OR Manager, Brown-Spath & Associates, and other groups. She writes the monthly "Quality-Cost Connection" column for *Hospital Peer Review* and serves as a quarterly guest columnist for *Hospital Case Management*.

Spath was awarded AHIMA's 1990 Literary Award and in 1998 was the winner of the AHIMA Legacy Award for her significant contributions to the health information management knowledge base through articles, chapters, books, and presentations. Spath can be contacted at patrice@brownspath.com.

The Contributors

. . . .

DIANE BOYNTON is director of human resource development at Central DuPage Health in Winfield, Illinois. Since joining Central DuPage Health in 1991, she has also worked with other health care organizations as a change management consultant through Gail Scott & Associates. Prior to her career in health care, she worked for ten years in the fields of school social work, crisis intervention, and community organization.

Boynton earned her bachelor of arts degree in sociology at Monmouth College in 1966 and a master of social work degree at the University of Kansas in 1975. She has published articles on change management, communication strategies, and leadership development. She has also served as faculty for the Institute for Healthcare Improvement's National Forums in 1995, 1996, and 1997 and is a member of the executive committee for the DuPage Education to Careers program.

GLORYANNE BRYANT has more than twenty-seven years of experience in the health information management profession. She currently serves as director of systemwide coding and HIM compliance for Catholic Healthcare West in San Francisco. In this role, Bryant is responsible for the coding compliance and education of forty-eight acute care facilities and a variety of other non-hospital-based health care entities in three states.

Bryant has conducted numerous ICD-9-CM and CPT-4 coding workshops for hospital-based coders. In addition, she has made an array of presentations on data quality, compliance, and documentation improvement to executives and health care administrators. She has been active in the California Health Information Association and is currently serving several national positions for the American Health Information Management Association.

JAMES B. CONWAY has served as chief operations officer of the Dana-Farber Cancer Institute since 1995. He holds a master of science degree from Lesley College, Cambridge, Massachusetts. He now serves on the adjunct faculty in the college's Graduate School of Management and in 1999 received the alumni's Community Service Award.

A diplomate of the American College of Healthcare Executives, Conway received the ACHE 1999 Massachusetts Regents Award as Healthcare Executive of the Year. He serves on the steering committee of the Massachusetts Coalition for the Prevention of Medical Errors and on the board of directors of the National Patient Safety Foundation. He is also a member of the physician issues advisory council of the Massachusetts Hospital Association, a member of the executive committee of the Medical, Academic and Scientific Community Organization (MASCO), and a longtime member of the board of the Ronald McDonald House in Boston.

CHRISTINA DEMPSEY is the nursing director for surgery at St. John's Regional Health Center in Springfield, Missouri. She earned her associate degree in nursing in 1985 from Missouri Southern State University and her bachelor of science degree in nursing from Southwest Missouri State University in Springfield, where she is currently pursuing a master's degree in business administration. Dempsey has worked in a number of clinical areas in her nursing career, including trauma, postanesthesia, intensive care, and surgery.

Dempsey is a certified operating room nurse (CNOR) and a member of the Association of Operating Room Nurses. She has served in the Association of Peri-Anesthesia Nurses (ASPAN); has written articles for *Breathline*, an ASPAN publication; and has been a speaker for ASPAN's international convention on such topics as interdepartmental cooperation and restructuring.

ANTHONY J. DIBELLA is an educator and thought leader in organizational learning and change management. He is president of Organizations Transitions, Inc., a consulting firm engaged in applied research and educational services, and adjunct professor of management at Worcester Polytechnic Institute. DiBella has analyzed company operations literally around the world and consulted with a wide range of organizations, including the Boston Management Consortium, Fidelity Investments, the Healthcare Forum, IBM Global Services, SAFECO insurance, the Uganda Central Credit Union, and the YMCA. He holds a doctoral degree from the Massachusetts Institute of Technology's Sloan School of Management and is the author of *How Organizations Learn* (Jossey-Bass, 1998) and *Learning Practices* (Prentice Hall, 2001). He can be reached via the World Wide Web at www.orgtransitions.com or via e-mail at ajdibella@orgtransitions.com.

CLAIRE R. DIXON-LEE is the president of MC Strategies, Inc. (www.mcstrategies.com). She is the former chair of the board of directors of the Joint Healthcare Information Technology Alliance (JHITA; www.jhita.org) and the former president of the American Health Information Management Association (AHIMA). She has over three decades of health information management experience and has worked for some of the industry's most distinguished technology companies in product design, data modeling, and dictionary development.

She has written numerous articles and presented seminars nationally and internationally on data quality, clinical documentation, regulatory issues, and computer-based patient records. Dixon-Lee holds a master's degree in medical epidemiology and a doctoral degree in public health policy and administration from the University of Illinois.

KATHLEEN J. HEERY is an experienced executive and manager in the areas of corporate education, training, and human resource development. She has created and implemented learning system infrastructures for a wide range of health care delivery systems. Currently she is a consultant to health care organizations in the areas of workforce development, communication practices, continuous learning environments, and the emerging world of health literacy and consumerism.

Heery holds a master's degree in communications and a bachelor's degree in English and writing; she is also a registered nurse. Her career spans twenty-five years in health care, with more than fifteen of them in corporate and executive positions at the national, regional, or local level. She has written many professional articles and has presented on a variety of subjects.

CONNIE E. KUYKENDALL is coordinator of nursing informatics at Union Hospital, Inc., in Terre Haute, Indiana. Her previous experience includes positions as supervisor of a medical and surgical floor, school nurse, coordinator of special projects, and acting administrative supervisor. She has been active in professional organizations and has held offices at various levels. She earned her bachelor's and master's degrees in nursing at Indiana State University and is currently working toward certification in nursing informatics.

MARY CAROLE MCMANN worked many years as a research dietitian and freelance medical writer before turning her skills to writing full time. While at Baylor College of Medicine, she coauthored five books in the popular Living Heart series. Since establishing Marimac Communications, Inc., in Houston, Texas, in 1996, she has written numerous projects both for the public and for physicians and other health professionals, many of which were approved for continuing medical education. Her professional publications include monographs, slide presentations, audio and video scripts, and journal articles; projects written for the public include brochures, articles for nationally distributed health newsletters, exhibit copy for the Museum of Health and Medical Sciences in Houston, and health-based Web site copy. She is author of the book *Soy Protein: What You Need to Know* (Avery, 2000) and coauthor of a soon-to-be-published book on orthostatic intolerance titled *The Fainting Phenomenon*. McCann can be contacted at MarimacComm@aol.com.

BRENDA I. MYGRANT works in the Continuing Medical Education Department of the Dannemiller Memorial Educational Foundation in San Antonio, Texas. She is responsible for numerous written projects and symposia for physicians and other health professionals with an emphasis on anesthesia and pain management. As an independent writer, she has also authored numerous projects for education of the general public as well as continuing medical education material for physicians and other health care professionals. Her publications include brochures, monographs, journal articles, abstracts, and research reports. During her twenty-year military career, Mygrant was the recipient of Tri-Service Nursing Research grants, served as principal investigator for studies on the effects of hydration and oxygenation on wound healing, and received the Evangeline Bovard Award for outstanding clinical nursing by a senior officer and the Army Legion of Merit. She can be contacted at BrendaM@pain.com.

PAMELA E. PAUSTIAN is an adjunct professor in the Healthcare Management and Information Sciences Division of the Department of Critical and Diagnostic Care, School of Health Related Professions, University of Alabama at Birmingham. She also is a full professor in the School of Business at Chadwick University. Her teaching assignments include ethics and law, organizational behavior, human resource management, operations management, and information systems applications in health care organizations.

In addition to traditional classroom and on-line instruction, Paustian provides corporate training in business microcomputer applications. She is experienced in the administrative and technical aspects of distance education as well as in instructional delivery using Internet technologies and consults to academic and professional organizations considering or implementing distance education programs. Her research interests include information system failures, managerial practices, and issues in distance education.

REBECCA PETERSEN is a registered nurse with a master's degree in health education. She began her clinical career as an emergency department staff nurse and then moved into management, directing the emergency departments at Alta Bates Medical Center in Berkeley for eighteen years and at Seton Medical Center in Daly City, California, for seven years. She assumed the directorship of the Hospital Consortium Education Network in 1995. Since then, she has grown the organization from five sponsoring hospitals to fifty-three hospitals plus Samuel Merritt College and the fire departments of Alameda County, California.

Petersen is president of the Society of Professionals in Healthcare and a member of the Association of California Nurse Leaders and the American Organization of Nurse Executives. She has given numerous presentations both locally and nationally for the American Hospital Association, Virginia Mason Distinguished Nurse Lecture Series, International Quality and Productivity Center, and other organizations. She can be contacted at becky@hospitalconsort.org.

DONALD C. SIBERY is president and chief executive officer of Central DuPage Health in Winfield, Illinois. He has worked in health care administration for more than twenty-eight years. From 1985 to

1996, he was president and CEO of Community Health Care, Inc., in Wausau, Wisconsin. He has served as executive vice president and CEO of Munson Medical Center in Traverse City, Michigan, and was the assistant director of professional services at Community Hospital in Indianapolis, Indiana.

Sibery earned his bachelor of arts degree at the University of Iowa in 1970 and a master of hospital administration degree at the University of Michigan in 1972. He is a fellow of the American College of Healthcare Executives.

DONNA J. SLOVENSKY is a professor at the University of Alabama, Birmingham, and director of its Bachelor of Science in Health Sciences program. She holds secondary appointments in the university's Department of Health Services Administration, Department of Management in the School of Business, Graduate School, and School of Medicine Center for Outcomes and Effectiveness Research and Education.

Slovensky's teaching assignments include strategic management, quality management, information management, competency assessment, and clinical outcomes evaluation. She also teaches doctoral seminars in strategic management and instructional methodologies for allied health educators, as well as corporate training courses.

Slovensky has consulting experience in a variety of health care organizations, including inpatient and ambulatory facilities, home health programs, and physician practices, in addition to consulting with HIM education programs. Her research interests include the strategic use of information resources, consumer and purchaser use of health provider outcomes information, and innovative teaching methodologies in health professions education.

ALICE T. SPEERS is an education specialist for perioperative services at William Beaumont Hospital, Royal Oak, Michigan. She is responsible for the development and evaluation of education programs for the operating room and acts as a consultant for the other programs provided by the department. In 1998, she received the Nightingale Award for Excellence in Nursing Education from Oakland University. She has extensive staff development experience in a variety of settings and has been a faculty member in a baccalaureate nursing program. She has published extensively on staff development and education topics.

RICHARD J. WAGNER is a professor of human resource management at the University of Wisconsin in Whitewater. His experience includes more than fifteen years as a corporate training director in a variety of organizational settings. He is active in consulting in the United States and Europe and has coauthored (with Robert Weigand) several articles on training evaluation and the book *Do It . . . and Understand! The Bottom Line on Corporate Experiential Learning* (Kendall/Hunt, 1994).

Wagner received his bachelor of science degree from Union College, his master of business administration degree from Gonzaga University, and his doctoral degree from Indiana University.

ROBERT WEIGAND is the director of management training and development at St. Luke's Hospital and Health Care Network in Bethlehem, Pennsylvania. His experience in health care spans two decades. He is also a part-time faculty member at several colleges, teaching psychology and business courses, and has coauthored (with Richard J. Wagner) several articles on training evaluation and the book *Do It . . . and Understand! The Bottom Line on Corporate Experiential Learning* (Kendall/Hunt, 1994).

Weigand received his bachelor of science degree in psychology from Ricker College and a master's degree in psychology from Assumption College.

KAREN L. ZAGLANICZNY is the director of education and research at William Beaumont Hospital and the program director of the Oakland University Beaumont Hospital graduate nurse anesthesia program. She also currently serves as chair of the American Association of Nurse Anesthetists (AANA). She is coeditor of the *Nurse Anesthesia* textbook and handbook (Harcourt Health Sciences, 2000) and of the *Clinical Guide to Pediatric Anesthesia* (Saunders, 1999) and is associate editor of the *AANA Journal*. She has lectured and published extensively on nurse anesthesia and related topics.

CHRISTINE S. ZAMBRICKI is assistant hospital director for the operating room, anesthesia, and perioperative services at William Beaumont Hospital, Royal Oak, Michigan. She is currently on the faculty at Oakland University and serves as an adviser to regulatory and accrediting bodies on many health care policy issues. She is past president of the American Association of Nurse Anesthetists and previously served as chair of the Michigan Board of Nursing.

SALLY ZUEL is director of education at Union Hospital, Inc., in Terre Haute, Indiana. Her previous experience includes positions as orientation coordinator, CPR coordinator, and staff and management positions in medical and surgical nursing. She is active in many professional organizations and serves on statewide committees for health care education. She earned her bachelor's and master's degrees in nursing at Indiana State University. She is certified in nursing administration and in nursing continuing education and staff development.

Guide to Effective Staff Development in Health Care Organizations

· ·

To Karen Fine,
my amazing and loving daughter and friend

Part I

. . . .

The Learning Imperative

· ·

Building the Context for Learning

An Executive Priority

Anthony J. DiBella

R ecently in a hospital near my home, a surgeon accidentally operated on the wrong child. A young girl, who was scheduled for reconstructive eye surgery, instead had her tonsils and adenoids removed, and tubes were placed in her ears. This case of mistaken identity apparently occurred when two girls of similar name and age were scheduled for outpatient surgery around the same time. According to a hospital spokesperson, "Words really can never express how devastated we all are, our worst nightmare" (Freyer, 2000).

As a participant in our modern health care system, do you ever stay up late at night wondering about this sort of trauma? Take consolation in the fact that such incidents occur infrequently. Yet according to a report from the Institute of Medicine (Kohn, Corrigan, and Donaldson, 2000), thousands of people die each year, and many others are injured because their medical caregivers made mistakes. Most mistakes occur not from the lack of basic or even advanced medical skills or training but from minor slip-ups such as misread handwriting or use of the wrong syringe.

There is a clear irony in many of the cases that are today considered medical accidents. When looked at from a historical perspective, modern medicine and its positive effects would have at one time been viewed as miraculous. Today's routine treatments for infections, cuts, and fractures and more dramatic interventions such as heart bypass surgery, organ transplantation, and in vitro fertilization are the result of a long series of lessons learned from experimentation and experience.

The health care industry has learned to innovate and improve its medical and administrative practices. Medical care is now available for a much more extensive set of problems among a greater number of patients. When mistakes happen, as can be expected in any complex system (Perrow, 1984), we wonder how such things like a misread medication order, mistaken surgery, or improper treatment can occur in these days of medical miracles. Just as the health care profession continues to learn about treating diseases, so must we learn how to reduce mistakes that end up harming patients.

Learning is, and always has been, an essential characteristic of health care services. By fostering learning among medical practitioners and the industry at large, health problems and conditions never before dealt with have become today's commonplace interventions. By nurturing a climate of trust and continual learning, health care leaders can create a context whereby errors are detected and corrected (Edmondson, 1996).

Learning is an essential element of a service system that seeks to continually expand its horizons and expectations. This chapter describes several important features of learning in organizations and the idiosyncratic aspects of health care as a learning system. The critical roles and tasks of health care leaders and managers in fostering a learning environment are presented. The information serves as a vital foundation for the remaining chapters in this book.

Learning Investments and Outcomes

A key aspect of American culture is a linear focus on short-term considerations (Hall, 1973). Investments such as time and financial resources are allocated on the basis of desired outcomes that can be quickly realized. As customers and stakeholders expect more and more and as the marketplace becomes ever more competitive, short-term performance drives many business decisions.

This has become as true for health care organizations as for other business enterprises. Change is occurring not solely because of cost pressures and the number of mergers and shifts in alliances between health care providers, health care institutions, and patients or customers but also because the very nature and definition of health care is being challenged. Whereas the health care industry was once dominated by a large number of nonprofit players, economic pressures are now expanding the for-profit dimension.

At the same time, questions are being raised about the core business of health care—are we in business to keep people healthy or to cure the sick? The issue here is whether health care has more of a reactive, curative role and responsibility or a proactive role to prevent illnesses from happening in the first place. These changes have resulted in a tremendous need for people and organizations to develop and increase learning capabilities.

Decisions to invest in learning test our cultural sense of priorities, values, and investment strategies. Learning has direct, short-term costs with an uncertain payoff. When we take time off to learn, we confront known production losses and unknown opportunity costs. Time lags between an investment in learning and realizing the rewards can be lengthy. When we acknowledge medical mishaps that can lead to learning, it's often detrimental to public relations and may expose us to legal liabilities. Yet organizations that fail to invest in learning lessen their ability to innovate, invent, or adapt to a changing environment. Change cannot occur unless we learn something new, even as we unlearn the old. While we may be reluctant to invest in learning, we clearly don't want to leave learning to chance or, even worse, to accept ignorance as the best way to compete or address life's medical challenges.

If life were ideal, we could rely on just-in-time learning. We would only spend time learning what we need when we needed it.

However, most learning is "just in case"; we learn something just in case we might need it. On airplanes, passengers are instructed in how to put on life vests with the hope that they will never have to do so. Fire departments guide the occupants of public buildings through exiting drills to prepare them for circumstances (an actual fire or bomb threat) that might require evacuation. Physicians learn about exotic or relatively unknown diseases in the event that such a case should someday present itself.

The option to learn does not represent much of a choice when so much is expected of us and when those expectations are getting higher. When we promote learning among our organizations and ourselves, our customers are happier, patients are healthier, employees are more productive, and our systems are more effective. One way to evaluate the need for learning investment is to consider a set of alternative outcomes: customers who complain, patients who experience poor quality of life, staff turnover, inefficient administration. We cannot put learning aside; if we do, we risk confronting such adverse consequences. Ultimately, they can mean closing the clinic's doors or failing to realize our true mission or vision like saving or extending life.

Historically, the individual has been the focus or target for learning; learning investments have been a key source of human capital development. Through what Peter Senge (1990) has called "personal mastery," each of us can learn and become proficient in some skill or ability. Most organizations, including those in health care, have focused on human resource development to help employees learn how to perform tasks or be effective in their jobs.

Yet as John Seeley Brown and Paul Duguid (2000) have explained, learning is fundamentally a social activity. We learn with and through others. On another level, the success of our health care system relies on a complex web of relationships between a diverse set of interdependent actors from researchers to caregivers to administrators. Learning occurs in and through this social network, and organizational success requires the interdependent learning of many (Goldratt and Cox, 1992). In effect, learning in organizations takes place on a level that transcends the individual actors. Learned expertise and capability are therefore the domain of the entire organization, not just of its individual members.

To ensure success, health care institutions must develop a learning capability that is independent of its individual members, who may come and go. The challenge is to share and then embed critical competencies so that they are an established part of the institution's way of doing things. A key task for managers and executives is to oversee and foster an environment in which learning may occur in the organizational systems for which they are accountable.

Learning in Health Care: Assets and Idiosyncrasies

One of the most stimulating aspects of working in different industries is confronting different situations, concerns, possibilities, and cultures. Every industry has distinctive features that facilitate or constrain learning. Learning activities that suit one industry don't work in another. When it comes to promoting learning (and change) in health care institutions, it is important to recognize both the facilitating and restraining forces.

Ten years ago, I codirected a research project on organizations as learning systems. One result was an integrative framework (DiBella and Nevis, 1998) that represented how and why team and organizational learning takes place. The generic framework, derived from case studies in a wide range of product and service companies, was designed for all sorts of social groupings, teams, and organizations in a variety of industries.

Subsequent research, funded by the Health Forum in San Francisco, looked at the idiosyncratic aspects of health care institutions as learning systems. The presumption up front was that health care is a unique industry and therefore the elements in our generic integrated framework would not be relevant to health care. What we found was that although there is overlap in how and why health care organizations and other organizations learn, there are several critical distinctions (Cavaluzzo, 1996).

These idiosyncrasies most likely stem from the nature of work performed by health care practitioners. There are significant and immediate implications of not learning or underperforming (a patient's loss of life or lower quality of life) that make learning an essential investment. For this reason, learning is a worthwhile and justifiable investment in health care. Also, when practitioners learn and apply new knowledge or skills, there is immediate feedback— the patient survives or quality of life improves. This feedback provides reinforcement and an intrinsic reward and motivation to the learner (Hackman and Oldham, 1980).

Learning Orientations

The more we know about and understand the dynamics of why and how learning occurs in organizations, the more we can do to promote learning. Rather than impose some theoretically derived notion or practice, managers can shape interventions that are consistent with the ways their organizations already learn or can be helped to learn. Our initial research generated a set of *learning orientations*, which represent processes whereby learning takes place and reflect the nature of what gets learned (DiBella and Nevis, 1998). Learning orientations are bipolar, linear, continuous dimensions that reflect contrasting approaches. Learning occurs all along the continuum; there is no right or wrong position. Polar extremes represent pure approaches to the same orientation; midpoints represent a balancing of approaches.

To examine learning processes in the context of health care, we conducted a series of in-depth field studies in six work settings in three health care systems. Through this process, we discovered that there are indeed some features of learning in health care organizations that are less significant in other industries. Differences occurred in how learning takes place but, more critically, also in why learning takes place and in the practices that promote learning. Our data prompted us to identify two learning orientations—*learning time frame* and *learning mode*—that represent essential distinctions in health care.

Learning Time Frame

Learning time frame is defined as "emphasis on learning that responds to immediate needs as compared to learning that may have long-term use." It can be represented as follows:

Learning Time Frame
Immediate .... **Long-term**

The two polar extremes (approaches) on the continuum of this learning orientation are "immediate" and "long-term." On one hand, some of the learning that takes place in health care contexts relates to capabilities that are used immediately in providing services to either diagnose or respond to health care concerns, especially emergencies. In health care, the effect of not learning (possible patient death) is so significant that professionals continually explore new technologies, procedures, and protocols of intervention. Service providers learn new tools and techniques because they are needed immediately to address or possibly rectify a condition that lacks a solution or is in need of a better one.

On the other hand, some learning in health care involves research to develop core competencies and capabilities over a longer term. Investments in the search for a cure for cancer, heart disease, new molecular compounds, the inner workings of cell development, and more efficient billing systems represent learning activities that have a long-term payoff. Health care providers must also promote learning to distinguish their values and contributions from competitors. Thus learning can also focus on the development of long-term advantages and strategic needs in order to survive in a competitive environment.

Learning Mode

A second essential learning orientation in health care is learning mode. This orientation is defined as "generating and sharing knowledge and skills through action or practice as compared to generating and sharing knowledge and skills through thinking or reflective activities." The two polar extremities (approaches) on this continuum are "experiential" and "cognitive":

Learning Mode

Experiential .... **Cognitive**

This learning orientation represents the necessity to learn new techniques in tacit form before they are thoroughly understood or can be made explicit.

In health care, there is a training tradition referred to as "see one, do one, teach one." Medical technology and procedures evolve so quickly that often there is little or no opportunity to specify how a procedure or protocol is done since it is entirely new or still evolving. In fact, it may have been used previously only in simulated situations with dummies, cadavers, or nonhuman subjects. Sometimes there is simply no way to learn about a procedure in an experimental way. You have to use the procedure on a real, live patient. For example, Dr. Michael DeBakey, the first physician to perform a human heart transplant, had tested the procedure on baboons and apes before applying his knowledge to a human subject. Even though DeBakey had conducted the transplant process several times in nonhuman subjects, when it came to actually doing the procedure with a live human being, there were still details he had to learn as he went through the experience.

Then, too, as much as medical care is constantly evolving, there is also a need for reflection and a thorough study of the advantages and disadvantages of different protocols and how they need to be used. Once an optimal solution has been identified and tested in clinical trials, it can be thoroughly documented. The explicit knowledge required to perform the procedure can then be embedded in a formal training program. This set of activities represents a cognitive learning approach in that knowledge and solutions to problems are generated and documented and can be studied prior to their ongoing use in a clinical setting. For example, the detailed procedure whereby the Food and Drug Administration approves drugs is an effort to learn cognitively to reduce any reliance on experiential learning.

Each of these two approaches to learning—experiential and cognitive—is used in health care. The need to take some action to cure or relieve the suffering of a sick patient will necessitate experiential learning given the risks involved. Yet the experience of dealing with many patients yields a set of cases that can be analyzed and used to develop cognitive learning that is then communicated formally outside of the demands and emergencies of a given situation.

Any health care organization can be typed on the basis of these two learning orientations, learning time frame and learning mode. Learning practices and processes reflect its relative emphasis on opposing approaches—immediate versus long-term, experiential versus cognitive. Different organizations are apt to value different priorities and practice different learning behaviors. Such differences would be reflected by typing at different points along the continua.

Learning Styles

Patterns or combinations or learning approaches reflect an organization's learning style (Shrivastava, 1983; DiBella, Nevis, and Gould, 1996). When we put several learning orientations together, we can create a composite picture of an organization's learning style. Much as individuals have different learning styles, so do organizations. Recognizing these styles can aid managers in determining how best to allocate resources to learning activities.

When the approaches of the two learning orientations are put into a matrix format, we can identify four distinctive learning styles (see Table 1.1). These styles are labeled *self-study*, *formal* (or *classroom*), *impromptu*, and *simulation*. Brief descriptions and examples of each of these styles follow.

Self-Study Learning

Self-study learning applies to approaches that are cognitive and immediate. It occurs when an individual must make immediate use of some established or known capability. A billing clerk who must learn how to process a patient's change of address goes to an administrative manual and reviews the formal procedure. A nurse who must learn whether there are adverse effects for a specific medication goes on-line to the manufacturer's Web site and reviews the documentation. A medical student discovers that a patient has symptoms suggestive of fibromyalgia and asks an instructor for more information about this condition. In these scenarios, the individual has an immediate need for learning about some problem or concern and then gathers information from sources of explicit knowledge.

Formal Learning

Formal learning reflects cognitive and long-term approaches. This style of learning is what medical education and practitioner training have traditionally involved. Explicit knowledge developed over time is packaged into coursework or training seminars. Practitioners attend to develop or update their skills or level of understanding. Through such investments, people come to understand

Table 1.1. Learning Styles as Represented by Learning Mode and Learning Time Frame.

Learning Mode	Learning Styles	
Cognitive	Self-Study	Formal (classroom)
Experimental	Impromptu	Simulation
	Immediate	Long-Term

Learning Time Frame

some principle or practice in the event that they confront circumstances requiring its use or application.

Impromptu Learning

Impromptu learning reflects approaches that are experiential and immediate. Impromptu learning occurs when there is inadequate knowledge to deal with a situation or when people lack the time to study or research what is already known. Health practitioners may confront emergent situations for which they have no training or novel circumstances that require adaptation of previous learning. In these cases, learning occurs simultaneously with the action. When Dr. DeBakey performed the first human heart transplant surgery, his learning in this situation was quite impromptu. Impromptu learning occurs whenever practitioners or administrators face new conditions, as during the development of cardiac stents, when new patient billing systems become operational, or when new therapies are used for the first time.

Simulation Learning

Simulation learning represents experiential and long-term approaches. Simulation learning occurs in more controlled circumstances when lessons and insights can emerge or be applied over a longer term. Lab experiments, cadaver work, clinical trials, and beta computer systems represent activities involving simulation. Errors and mistakes can occur, be detected, and responded to without worry or fear of immediate consequences.

Implications of Learning Styles

Our research indicated that all these learning styles were being used in the different contexts we studied. Some organizations exhibited behaviors that suggested they had a dominant style, while others exhibited a broader emphasis on all the styles. The relative dominance of a learning style reflects the nature of the work context and the demands placed on staff. For example, in research centers, we see learning activities typical of a long-term approach, and in hospitals, we find activities typical of an immediate approach.

Rather than emphasize a singular approach or style, managers would do better to support a diversity of styles. In effect, organizations can be viewed as having a portfolio of styles. Those with a broader portfolio are apt to have multiple competencies and a greater ability to adapt to change than organizations that rely on a single style.

By focusing on an organization's learning portfolio in its entirety, managers can stop wondering about the right learning style and start thinking about how to complement the various styles that exist across the entire health care system. A critical role of health care executives is to allocate learning resources to activities that reflect these different styles. Such an allocation should be consistent with the mission, vision, and culture of the institution. Learning activities should be evaluated and supported because they fit the style or styles of the organization rather than because they were found in some benchmarking study. Best practices that suit one organization's context (and its learning portfolio) may fail miserably in another organization (DiBella, 2001).

Facilitating Factors

Learning orientations represent a descriptive side of learning; our research indicated that there is also a normative side. Learning is more apt to occur when certain conditions are in place. Such conditions, which we have called *facilitating factors*, promote specific types of learning and directly affect the speed whereby learning occurs. When facilitating factors are weak, learning either does not occur, occurs quite slowly, or is irrelevant to the mission of the organization.

Our research found high overlap between the facilitating factors in non-health-related industries and the factors or practices that promote learning in health care. In a few cases, we had to adapt definitions and labels because of the idiosyncrasies of the health care industry lexicon. The most critical change pertained to a facilitating factor we had labeled *climate of openness*, defined as "open communications among organizational members where problems or errors are shared, not hidden." To health care staff, this factor isn't about openness; it's about relationships between people and the feeling they have for one another. To health care practitioners, this factor became known as *trusting relationships*, defined as "the amount of trust and open communication between members and the respect that team members had for mutual growth and development." For health care professionals, this was the single most important facilitating factor that caused learning to occur. Basically, when you trust your colleagues, you can be open about sharing not only your successes but also your failures (Edmondson, 1996). Within that context of support and mutual respect, a person can take risks to learn, realizing that colleagues will appreciate the effort even though the learning may fall short of its goal.

In analyzing why learning took place in health care, three other essential facilitating factors were identified: *learning confidence, shared vision,* and *learning enjoyment.*

Learning Confidence

Learning confidence is defined as "experience in learning from successes, mistakes, and specific events; experience in trying new things; the belief that all groups can learn." In effect, learning confidence represents historical precedent: if you have learned in the past, you are apt to have confidence that you can learn in the present. This factor reflects a person's skill in addressing an area of unknown competency with conviction and confidence that the skill can be acquired and learned. And the more one has done of this in the past, the more one is apt to do it in the present. Subsequent independent research has confirmed the value of this facilitating factor in health care (Bohmer, Edmondson, and Pisano, forthcoming). Learning confidence allows people working in health care to embrace new protocols and techniques and put them into practice.

Consider, for example, the frequency with which organ transplant and heart bypass procedures are done today. Only a select group of surgeons performed these procedures at first. However, many other surgeons with learning confidence have since acquired this skill.

Shared Vision

A second facilitating factor that is key to promoting learning in the context of health care is shared vision. Readers of Peter Senge's work will not be surprised by this addition, since it is one of his five critical disciplines that promote learning (Senge, 1990). Shared vision is defined as "shared understanding of and commitment to the creation of a desired future." The notion of shared vision is critical in health care because of the historical focus on service to community and humankind. Whereas certain industries have adopted the vision of profitability, the health care industry has traditionally considered its mission one of excellence in patient care. Learning in health care occurs because the people share the same values and vision as the organization.

Learning Enjoyment

To anyone who remembers the movie and television program *MASH*, it will come as no surprise that learning enjoyment is a facilitating factor. The pace of change in health care and the critical demands to do things exactly right create an environment in which coping mechanisms are essential. Learning enjoyment is "celebrating learning achievements and creating an atmosphere where humor and fun are part of the process of acquiring new knowledge." Failures and mistakes are life-and-death matters in health care practice, and unless some humor and lightness can be brought to the sharing of such occurrences, there is apt to be little sharing of the lessons learned. Humor is a crucial coping mechanism. It adds to the playful mode of inquisitiveness and allows for the open sharing of information.

Management's Role in Promoting Learning

The learning orientations and facilitating factors identified in our research reflect the unique and essential aspects of health care that influence learning. A key question is, What does it all mean for the health care executive? How can leaders ensure that learning will be pursued in the most effective manner?

The main responsibility of any executive is to set the vision for some work team or the organization as a whole. The executive must then manage ongoing activities, change, or adaptations in the direction of that vision. Leading health care demands good management; even as good management requires good leadership. In today's environment of continuous change, learning capability is a necessary skill that keeps organizations moving toward their vision. Five actions can guide health care executives in promoting learning in their organizations:

1. Inventory existing learning practices.

2. Determine strategic knowledge needs.

3. Shape the context and climate for learning.

4. Provide adequate resources.

5. Participate in learning collaborations.

Inventory Existing Learning Practices

Before jumping into action to create learning organizations, executives would be better served by taking an organization development approach, of which the first step is to inventory existing learning (DiBella, 2001). Many learning organization initiatives have failed because they overlook current learning practices and try to impose specific learning behaviors or best practices that are at variance with established ones. In effect, managers need be mindful of what presently exists in the learning portfolio of their work teams or organizations. Managers should be aware of the learning approaches and styles exhibited by their organizations. Top executives should employ a systems perspective to acknowledge the relative emphasis of different learning styles such as self-study, formal, impromptu, and simulation.

Determine Strategic Knowledge Needs

While acknowledging and appreciating the learning styles currently employed in the organization, managers must determine whether those styles produce the learning and knowledge required to achieve the organization's vision and strategic goals. Otherwise, the learning that takes place will not be aligned with the knowledge needs or task demands placed on the organization. To determine knowledge needs requires, of course, some explicit strategy that serves as a guide to realizing the organization's mission. With that in hand, an executive can ask: Given the different components of our strategy, what needs to be learned, who needs to learn what, and how will that learning take place? Appropriate action plans can then be established.

Shape the Context and Climate for Learning

When learning is an essential aspect of work, managers must shape the context whereby learning styles can be effectively employed. The more supportive the context for learning, the more apt it is to occur. In health care, this means emphasizing specific facilitating factors. First, practitioners need to feel that they function in a network of trusting relationships in which they feel safe enough to report errors and mistakes so that everyone can learn from them. The reporting of errors spawns learning opportunities and builds learning confidence. Finally, organizations need a context where learning enjoyment can diffuse the tension surrounding the personal struggles and family dramas that are so much a part of health care. In a supportive environment, the failures of experience can more readily be converted to lessons learned.

Provide Adequate Resources

Nearly everyone agrees that learning is desirable until the time comes for allocating resources—time, space, money, and personnel. It's easier to talk about the need for learning than it is to commit the resources required to make learning happen. As discussed earlier, learning is an investment in some future outcome whose value is often not easy to envision or quantify. Investing in learning means that fewer resources can be allocated to short-term productive activities, and that is difficult to do when immediate results appear more rewarding. Learning won't just happen; it must be nurtured with resources. Managers must make resources available to generate opportunities for creating and building knowledge. Such commitment also has symbolic value. When executives allocate funds for training, allow time for debriefings, and reward staff for reporting and learning from mistakes instead of covering them up, they demonstrate that organizational improvement is not just rhetoric.

Participate in Learning Collaborations

One cost-effective and often overlooked learning activity is corporate communities of practice. In these institutional collaborations, organizations share the costs and benefits of major learning initiatives. The notion of communities of practice customarily refers to social groups that informally produce learning for their members (Wenger, 1998). Alliances have become a common part of health care, as evidenced by the way in which individual physicians and providers have organized themselves into groups for business purposes. For many years, health care institutions have joined together to develop (that is, learn) solutions to health care problems that require a level of investment beyond the capability of any one organization. Corporate communities of practice, like the Health Forum and the Institute for Healthcare Improvement, provide an opportunity for participants to develop and share medical innovations. Some collaborations involve private health care organizations alone; others involve public organizations or private foundations. Executives should make participating in these alliances an integral part of their learning strategy.

Learning: An Investment in the Future

Most of us believe or know the value of learning, but many of us are reluctant to invest the time or money that is required. The health care executive and manager must legitimate the need for learning and promote the conditions that are essential for learning to occur. Perhaps the greatest challenge is that some learning takes place only after we acknowledge our mistakes and faults. This places into opposition the need for a manager to support and show appreciation for current efforts while at the same time encouraging staff to learn and attain higher levels of performance and effectiveness. In effect, managers must be both cheerleaders (to appreciate, encourage, and reward) and critics (to point out shortfalls in performance). Leading medical care successfully confronts the demands of these oppositional roles.

Health care organizations are being subjected to ongoing changes in technology and consumer interests and preferences. While training activities help personnel develop specific skills to meet today's work demands, learning capability helps organizations adapt to the ongoing changes. The health care leaders and executives who focus on learning are making an investment in their organizations' future. True success comes from emphasizing both short-term operational considerations and long-term development ones. Health care leaders must creatively meet the demands of these complementary priorities.

References

Bohmer, R. M., Edmondson, A. C., and Pisano, G. P. "Managing New Technology in Medicine." In R. Herzlinger (ed.), *Consumer-Driven Health Care*. San Francisco: Jossey-Bass, forthcoming.

Brown, J. S., and Duguid, P. *The Social Life of Information*. Boston: Harvard Business School Press, 2000.

Cavaluzzo, L. "Enhancing Team Performance." *Health Forum Journal*, 1996, 39(5), 59–61.

DiBella, A. J. *Learning Practices: Assessment and Action for Organizational Improvement*. Upper Saddle River, N.J.: Prentice Hall, 2001.

DiBella, A. J., and Nevis, E. C. *How Organizations Learn: An Integrated Strategy for Building Learning Capability*. San Francisco: Jossey-Bass, 1998.

DiBella, A. J., Nevis, E. C., and Gould, J. M. "Understanding Organizational Learning Capability." *Journal of Management Studies*, 1996, 33, 361–379.

Edmondson, A. C. "Learning from Mistakes Is Easier Said Than Done: Group and Organizational Influences on the Detection and Correction of Human Error." *Journal of Applied Behavioral Science*, 1996, 32(1), 5–28.

Freyer, F. J. "Hasbro Doctor Operates on Wrong Child in ID Mixup." *Providence Journal*, Dec. 23, 2000, p. 1.

Goldratt, E., and Cox, J. *The Goal: A Process of Ongoing Improvement*. (2nd ed.) Great Barrington, Mass.: North River Press, 1992.

Hackman, R. J., and Oldham, G. R. *Work Redesign*. Boston: Addison-Wesley, 1980.

Hall, E. T. *The Silent Language*. New York: Anchor Books, 1973.

Kohn, L.T., Corrigan, J. M., and Donaldson, M. S. (eds.). *To Err Is Human: Building a Safe Health System*. Washington, D.C.: National Academy Press, 2000.

Perrow, C. *Normal Accidents: Living with High-Risk Technologies*. New York: Basic Books, 1984.

Senge, P. *The Fifth Discipline: The Art and Practice of the Learning Organization*. New York: Doubleday, 1990.

Shrivastava, P. "A Typology of Organizational Learning Systems." *Journal of Management Studies*, 1983, 20, 7–28.

Wenger, E. *Communities of Practice: Learning, Meaning, and Identity*. Cambridge: Cambridge University Press, 1998.

2

. . . .

An Organizational Model for Continuous Learning

Kathleen J. Heery

Constant change and turmoil within the health care industry places many new demands on health care executives. Higher performance outputs, efficient practices, and bottom-line effectiveness are required at all levels of patient care delivery. However, workforce issues have become barriers to achieving these goals. Many health care employees are nearing retirement, and staffing shortages are threatening the stability of patient services. Added to these workforce issues are the challenges of decreased reimbursements, increased regulatory requirements, and aging populations that require more health care services. This unprecedented collision of demographics and economics has created a climate in which health care organizations must make a strategic investment in workforce training in order to survive.

Although factors such as reimbursement rates and regulations are beyond the immediate control of health care executives, many of the structural and environmental circumstances that affect the workforce can be effectively managed. A solid performance management system and a continuous learning infrastructure help the organization retain competent employees. These factors are also key recruitment tools. Work environments are known to directly influence employee retention. Studies show that lack of recognition and career development is the most common reason why employees leave organizations (Watson Wyatt Worldwide, 2000; Kaye and

Evans, 2000; American Society of Training and Development, 2000).

A Learning Climate

Human resource practices, career management programs, training initiatives, and collaborative education partnerships are key components of an organization's commitment to continuous learning. However, merely having these elements in place is not enough. These systems and processes must be supported by a climate that encourages employees to share innovations and practices. In a learning organization, acquisition of new knowledge and skills must be ongoing and not merely a onetime event. Targeted outcomes help employees transfer knowledge into practice. In support of this process, the organization must create the structure, communication links, and resource systems that are necessary to expand clinical excellence.

Learning organizations ensure that employees know what adds value to the health care delivery system. Unfortunately, training practices in many health care organizations are often obsolete and do not meet the educational needs of increasingly large and diverse workforces. Shifting care delivery environments and changing work roles are challenging the traditional employee training systems in many organizations.

Therefore, changes are needed in four areas of workforce development: linkage with organizational goals, systems in human resource and performance management, infrastructure for training and development practices, and collaborative educational partnerships. Defining and linking these systems and functions creates an organizational model for continuous learning.

The Hierarchical and Environmental Learning Partnership (HELP) model produces strategic and operational plans as well as staffing and learning plans that create continuous learning climates. These plans and their subsequent implementation form a systematic and systemic model for performance excellence. Exhibit 2.1 illustrates this model in greater detail.

Exhibit 2.1. Hierarchical and Environmental Learning Partners (HELP) Model for Continuous Learning Organizations.

Strategic Plan

Analyze business environment, major initiatives, critical success factors (CSF).

Explore and determine target service or product markets.

Set mission, vision, and goals.

Operational Plans

Define services along product or service line strategies linked to business goals.

Translate strategy into daily actions that align with CSF.

Establish and implement guidelines, workflow, and evaluation systems.

Staffing and Workforce Plan

Define performance standards linked to business goals and CSF.

Define and implement recruitment and retention strategy.

Establish performance and evaluation metrics that measure CSF outputs.

Training and Learning Plan

Establish data-driven learning systems linked to business goals and CSF.

Create learning and curriculum infrastructure linked to performance goals.

Establish various partnerships to leverage resources.

In a continuous learning environment, performance systems and learning initiatives are linked to business goals. However, many conventional training systems in health care organizations do not make these connections. Workforce factors are handled in a different manner. The important differences between traditional training systems and continuous learning systems are summarized in Table 2.1.

It is evident that training system transformations must take place to support a learning environment. The benefits of these changes are detailed in the last column in Table 2.1. The continuous learning system practices that organizations must adopt are described in greater detail later in this chapter.

Linkage with Organizational Goals

People working in high-performing organizations have an understanding of the vision and business goals that must be translated into operational reality all the way down the line. According to Peter Senge (1990), shared vision binds people together around a common identity, confers a sense of destiny, and gives coherence to diverse activities within the organization.

The chief executive officer shapes the organization's learning climate. Through the development of a shared vision and the business strategies that support this vision, the CEO can affect the destiny of education and training activities. Just as strategy is set for finance, operations, and marketing, it must also be set for training and learning.

Strategic objectives for workforce education must be linked to the organization's mission, core business initiatives, and critical success factors (CSF). Without such a linkage, there is no guarantee that resource-intensive employee training activities will actually help the organization achieve its business goals.

The model in Exhibit 2.2 illustrates the relationship of a strategic goal with workforce training requirements. Achievement of strategic goals often requires new workforce competencies or reinforcement of existing skills (or both). Learning systems must expand to educate and support team efforts as well as individual learning needs. By planning for the training needs associated with each strategic goal, the organization can integrate learning opportunities into its training system. Thus the organization can ensure that its workforce is prepared keep up with the ever-changing tasks that need to be performed.

Another critical element needed for effective workforce training is the strategy for information technology (IT). Technology

Exhibit 2.2. Relationship Between Strategic Goals and Workforce Training Requirements.

Strategic goal: To expand women's health services

↓

Performance goal: To increase outpatient revenue for women's health services by 20 percent

↓

Major operational initiatives:
• Create new women's health clinic
• Expand and strengthen postpartum home care services
• Expand family-centered maternity unit
• Identify and implement relevant educational programs for the community

↓

Strategic training objectives:
• Improve the ability of our workforce to provide competent, family-centered maternity care
• Raise awareness of women's health issues and articulate the benefits of women's health services to the public
• Establish and maintain the center as a patient and consumer education resource for physicians, departments, and other affiliates

Table 2.1. Comparison of Traditional Training Systems and Continuous Learning Systems.

Critical Workforce Factors	Traditional Training Systems	Continuous Learning Systems	Benefits of Continuous Learning Systems
Linkage with organizational goals	Work practices and learning systems are not linked to the organization's mission, vision, or core business initiatives. Leadership is unaware of or uninformed about the organization's workforce development and learning systems, training strategies, and practices.	Workforce practices and learning systems are linked to the organization's mission and core business initiatives. Leadership has created a learning structure that supports workforce development and learning systems, training strategies, and practices.	• Senior management support gives credibility to system efforts. • Work practices support organization critical success factors. • Workforce development and learning is more responsive to organizational needs. • Validated performance issues are addressed.
Human resource and performance management	Focus is on job descriptions, tasks, and procedures without defined departmental or organization performance outputs. Emphasis is on recruitment, not retention. Managers focus on improving individual performance rather than on improving the systems in which individuals work. Managers have little or no training in how to improve systems.	Focus is on matching position responsibilities to organizational needs through identified performance outputs. Emphasis is on retention as well as recruitment. Managers focus on fixing systems and eliminating barriers. Managers have leadership support and training for their ongoing responsibilities.	• Accountability of the human resource department is improved. • Employee productivity is increased. • Staff retention is improved. • Success is measured against defined performance outputs. • Managers have the training and tools needed to be more effective. • Learning structure meets accreditation and regulatory mandates. • Employees are recognized for contributions made in achieving organizational goals.

Training and development	Internal trainers create learning programs that are often disconnected from operational goals and employee career needs. There is little to no relationship between learning systems, performance improvement, and competency programs. Training professionals use an outdated staff education model.	The training infrastructure is linked to human resource functions and operational goals. Employees are supported at all levels of the organization. More structured "just-in-time" resources are available at the point of service delivery. Employees quickly transfer training into practice. Training professionals function as performance consultants and learning advisers.	• Nonrelevant training programs are eliminated, and costs are reduced. • Training responds to actual performance needs. • Learning systems improve productivity and decrease costs. • Access to learning resources in practice areas is improved. • Employee involvement in training opportunities is increased.
Partnerships	There are few or no partnerships with area or regional schools, workforce development boards, or other learning vendors.	Local and regional educational resources are leveraged to produce cost savings, better-trained workers, and targeted outcomes.	• The health care organization is no longer competing with educational groups, which reduces training costs. • The ability to establish internships and programs to address clinical shortage areas is increased. • Duplication and redundancy are decreased by tapping into other training resources. • Systems are established to "grow" the organization's own employees in key shortage areas.

continues to play an increasingly pivotal role in learning and training design.

Linking strategic plans with organizational training needs is the
crucial first step toward building a high-performance learning organization.

Human Resource and Performance Management

Human resource management produces the overall structure for
continuous learning environments. The organization must create
a strategic workforce and staffing plan that examines current and
future personnel needs and also defines employee performance
measures. A learning infrastructure will be successful only if
employees and managers are aware of performance expectations.
Training and development activities should be part of the human
resource function.

The workforce and staffing plan drives the organization's workforce development system. The plan serves as a guide for position
and competency development, career management, performance
measurement, and recruitment and retention.

Position and Competency Development

Advances in technology, mergers, and other factors can change
job responsibilities overnight. Human resource and operations managers must work together to ensure that descriptions of job functions are current and accurate. Common language should be used
to describe job performance criteria. These criteria must include
clear expectations, minimum and desired performance standards,
associated competencies, defined performance outputs, and reward
systems. These criteria provide targeted goals for training and specific guidelines for performance evaluations.

A careful analysis of expected performance outputs and position
competencies provides an overall framework for the organization's
hiring and evaluation systems. Performance standards must support
organizational goals. Competencies are measurable outputs that

describe behaviors needed to meet performance standards. Though performance standards can be similar across job families, competencies vary from role to role. It is crucial to define and develop key competencies for employees so that the organization spends it training and development dollars efficiently.

Compensation and pay-for-performance systems then reward crucial performance outputs defined at the department, team, or individual level. As health care systems continually transform, increasing emphasis on multidisciplinary and cross-departmental projects requires more team-focused reward and recognition systems. In this environment, performance expectations often center on systemic problem solving, use of best practices, and the transfer of learning and knowledge into practice.

Performance outputs align with the organization's critical success factors to keep them on target. Outputs can be measured through performance metrics that evaluate productivity for teams or departments. These metrics must be clearly delineated and communicated to individuals to enable them to see how their role supports these goals. The model in Exhibit 2.3 demonstrates the relationship of an organizational goal to individual competencies and performance expectations at the department level.

Career Management

A functional career management system helps attract, retain, sustain, and "grow your own" employees—a practice adopted by many organizations as a way of increasing the available number of qualified workers. Career management systems include initiatives such as a career ladder program that helps employees identify and obtain the skills necessary for advancement. The preset career-path models of yesterday are being replaced by employee development guidance systems that link performance goals and core competencies.

A functional career management system should assist employees in attaining their personal mastery level. As defined by Senge (1990), personal mastery is another essential cornerstone of

Exhibit 2.3. Position Performance Criteria for a Registration Clerk.

Strategic organization goal: To decrease risk by creating and implementing an organizationwide corporate compliance program

↓

Operational plan: Create and implement the organization's code of conduct

↓

Performance standard (individual or team): Practices and adheres to all standards outlined in organization's code of conduct

↓

Competencies (behaviors specific to registration clerk):
• Consistently inputs patient data according to defined departmental procedures
• Consistently ensures confidentiality and privacy of all patient information
• Reports significant policy and procedural variations to supervisor within twenty-four hours

↓

Performance metrics (department or organization):
• Increase registration accuracy by 15 percent
• Decrease coding errors by 10 percent
• Decrease financial risk to organization

learning organizations. Career management programs support personal mastery through the use of various communication channels, career centers, coaching and mentoring, and learner-centered training programs.

The career management systems should align employee wants with organization needs. This is a key strategy for attracting difficult-to-recruit employees. For example, a long-term care facility in New

England implemented a pilot career ladder program for certified nursing assistants (CNAs). A year later, CNA retention rates were 74 percent (up from 20 percent), and the facility no longer had to hire temporary agency staff to fill CNA vacancies (an annual savings of $500,000). This example illustrates how an investment in the workforce can yield financial gains for the organization.

Performance Measurement

The employee appraisal system in a learning organization measures an individual or team's contribution to business goals and critical success factors. Performance measurement is not a onetime event. It is a system of ongoing observation, assessment, and evaluation that promotes goal achievement and production of targeted outcomes.

Organization outcomes are produced through workflow processes and systems, and employees are rewarded or refocused on the basis of their contributions. The performance review examines each employee's contribution to his or her department's goals and any specific project goals that support critical organizational initiatives.

However, not everything needs to be measured—only those activities and outputs critical to the organization's success. For example, to implement a corporate compliance program, all employees must be trained in the organization's code of conduct and also shown how their job responsibilities support the compliance program objectives. The information in Exhibit 2.3 illustrates how the hospital registration clerk's individual performance supports both department and organization compliance goals.

Recruitment and Retention

An organization's recruitment and retention plan encompasses all of the abovementioned workforce development systems. Defined roles and competencies, internal systems for advancement, and clear performance standards will help in recruiting new employees and retaining those already in your workforce. A comprehensive workforce development strategy will position your organization as the preferred employer.

Employees that feel valued and challenged by an organization are more likely to stay working for that organization. When leaders provide employees with a variety of learning options that help them achieve professional and personal goals, the organization has a higher rate of employee retention. Find out why employees leave your organization. Exit interviews should be conducted and the results used to improve retention strategies. All too often health care organizations spend more time and money on recruitment activities than they do on employee retention.

Organizations find that investing in the human resource management function in the interest of creating a healthy environment is well worth the price. Such an investment is the second step toward building a high-performance learning organization.

The Training and Development Plan

The organization's plan for employee training and development draws from the information and goals expressed in the workforce and staffing plan. The training plan defines the organization's learning strategy and details the learning tools and options that help employees obtain and retain skills and knowledge.

The training process itself can be organized in a number of ways. However, it is important to have seamless links between the human resource and training functions. This collaboration forms a foundation for learning systems that creates and sustains continuous learning environments. There are four key elements of an efficient and effective learning system: performance improvement, data-driven training, flexible learning opportunities, and outcomes evaluation.

Performance Improvement

Learning systems must shift their traditional focus on training to a focus on performance. To achieve this shift, training professionals should partner with operations managers to match training initiatives and learning outcomes with the skills needed to perform job responsibilities. With the shelf life of new knowledge growing shorter and job positions changing almost overnight, the training imparted to the health care workforce must constantly evolve to meet new demands.

Learning systems must help people identify and correct performance deficits, adopt or establish best practices, and monitor learning outputs based on actual data and performance gaps. Ideal learning systems provide a mix of formal training programs and e-learning tactics that give employees "just-in-time" access to the information they need to do their jobs. All too often the traditional learning systems in health care organizations fail to realize these ideals. Consider the learning system in your organization. Does it

- Provide workforce training that helps achieve expected business results?

- Adequately prepare the workforce for job responsibility transitions?

- Measure specific learning outcomes that are linked to required competencies?

- Measure critical areas vital to the organization's strategic initiatives?

- Create flexible learning opportunities for employees?

- Help managers and staff identify knowledge deficits?

- Adequately meet the needs of all workers, not just the nursing staff?

- Provide interdisciplinary programs that encourage disciplines to approach patient care as a team?

- Help people transfer knowledge into practice?

- Make information and learning available where and when employees need it?

- Provide for creation and oversight of knowledge management?

- Provide a variety of learning options for all levels of staff?

- Leverage technology and e-learning strategies?

- Identify and partner with appropriate colleges and learning institutions?

- Offer learning tools that are developed jointly by training professionals and trainees?

If you answered no to any of the questions, your learning system is probably disconnected from operational needs and producing less than optimal results.

Transitioning your learning system will require a shift in design and instruction approaches. Many organizations have started using performance and learning advisers. These consultants serve as knowledge managers, using the organization's strategic goals and performance data to develop learning responses.

Managing Knowledge Capital

Health care is a service industry that depends on its employees' knowledge to be successful. That's why management of knowledge capital is so important. Knowledge management connects the information seekers with the knowledge holders. To effectively manage the organization's collective knowledge, there must be systems that allow employees to access meaningful information where they need it and when they need it. Consider this scenario: A nurse is troubleshooting problems with a new piece of equipment at 2:00 A.M. She cannot wait for the next training class one week away. She needs information and answers right now. The learning organization provides this nurse with on-the-spot access to self-learning tools. Intranet training programs, informational databases, and speakers' bureaus are three examples of integrated knowledge systems that help support the workforce in a learning organization.

Within the organization, structured knowledge is translated into training programs and databases. However, unstructured knowledge is often scattered throughout the organization in e-mails, publications, and employees' heads (Bantleman, 2000). One way to bring these two assets together is through better management of your organization's various knowledge resources. Employees, information professionals, managers, training instructors, and human resource staff must work together to identify sources of structured and unstructured knowledge. The next step is to create improved knowledge-sharing opportunities for continuous learning.

Continuous Learning and Practice

Learning opportunities and training must be available where most needed—at the point of service delivery. When knowledge acquisition occurs almost simultaneously with application, employees have an opportunity to use this knowledge in their work areas. It is generally agreed that learning should be put into practice as quickly as possible to increase knowledge retention. An employee's rate of knowledge retention drops 25 percent the first week following a training program and then falls off significantly after that (Muirio, 2000).

Using new technologies, health care organizations can create learning communities. E-learning systems allow employees to search, access, and retrieve specific knowledge they need for immediate use on the job. Content should be focused and distilled to its bare essentials. The goal should be to impart "need to know" rather than "nice to know" information.

Data-Driven Training

In a continuous learning environment, the education department offers structured training programs that are linked to the organization's core operational needs. For example, if the organization has a commitment to workforce career management, training and development programs are designed to complement this strategy. Employees are taught how to remain competent in current roles and also how to advance into other positions that might be needed to achieve the organization's business goals.

Educational interventions should be considered only after careful study of employee training needs. For example, a patient accounts manager in a hospital asked the training department to conduct a diagnosis and procedure coding class for employees to help correct billing errors. When the problem was analyzed in greater detail, it was found that the billing problems were not due to a lack of knowledge on the part of the billing clerks. The errors were actually caused by data entry inconsistencies in the patient registration process. Coding instruction for the billing clerks would not have solved the problem, since it originated with the registration process. When training staff function as performance consultants and learning advisers, instead of "old-style" educators, the causes of problems are investigated so that appropriate actions can be taken.

Many data sources are used to select training program topics, including patient and employee surveys, needs assessments, quality monitoring reports, patient complaints, productivity reports, and safety audits. The information derived from these sources forms the basis for training priorities in the organization. Sources of unstructured knowledge are often the products of various projects within the organization. Lessons learned, templates, and reports are all examples of useful data available to share with employees.

Only through the analysis of information can the organization be sure that its workforce is learning necessary skills. Employees must be good at what they do, and what they do must in the best interests of the organization (Senge, 2000).

Flexible Learning Opportunities

A learning organization does not rely on only one method for training employees. A variety of learning opportunities are offered. Traditional classroom-style training can be very expensive, and many organizations are replacing it with self-directed learning systems. One small 180-bed hospital found that it was spending $80,000 a year to conduct mandatory eight-hour classroom-style education programs for the nursing staff. By shifting this training to self-learning systems, the hospital saved $40,000 in direct labor costs and increased productivity by sixteen hundred hours per year. Self-directed learning systems can take many forms. Various types of systems are described in other chapters in this book.

Outcomes Evaluation

Too often training departments measure inputs instead of outputs. Inputs are generally utilization measures such as number of classes and average attendance. Outputs are measures of results, such as what people learned and how the new knowledge affected job performance. While it is necessary to track attendance and program integrity, a learning organization doesn't rely solely on input data to determine the value of training. An effective learning system integrates performance standards, learning outcomes, and performance metrics. Table 2.2 illustrates this relationship for the registration clerk position. Satisfactory achievement of the performance standard is based in part on the employee's ability to demonstrate specific learning outcomes. An employee may actually have the knowledge to perform a function but is unable to apply that knowledge due to a system or process problem. Ensuring learning outcomes helps determine performance problems at the system, process, or person level.

Table 2.2. Relationship Among Performance Standards, Learning Outcomes, and Performance Metrics.

Performance Standard	Learning Outcome	Performance Metrics
Practices and adheres to all standards outlined in the organization's code of conduct	• Demonstrates the ability to enter data and information accurately into computer systems • States methods for reporting variances to supervisor according to policy outlined in code of conduct • Completes all required compliance training programs and processes (initial and ongoing)	• Performance evaluations are satisfactory. • Registration is accurate and complete within the 90 percent threshold.

Another method to evaluate training investment outputs is for your organization to participate in benchmarking activities. Each year, the American Society for Training and Development (ASTD) conducts a survey of organizations that results in a "state of the industry" training benchmarking report. This report collects information from all types of organizations in the following areas:

• Training expenditures and practices

• Organizational performance

• Learning technologies

• Use of providers and evaluation

• Salaries and functioning of internal training staff

• Intellectual capital measures

• Customer service practices

This survey allows organizations to benchmark their training performance and outputs against other training department activities both within and outside the health care industry. For more information about this benchmarking survey, visit the ASTD Web site (www.astd.org) or call (800) 628-2783.

Partnerships

Alexis Herman (2000), former U.S. secretary of labor, described the country's labor issues as more of a "skills" shortage than a worker shortage, citing millions of potential but untapped workers. However, these millions of untapped workers come with a plethora of learning needs.

Health care organizations are ill prepared to meet the learning needs of these workers, yet they must tap into this labor pool to fill many emerging job positions. To ensure that skilled health care workers are available for hire, the training and development department in health care organizations must establish partnerships with regional colleges and training vendors. These partners can assist health care employers in building workforces for the future and meeting the continuing education needs of current employees.

Is your internal training and development program unnecessarily duplicating what is already available outside of your facility? Local colleges and universities, area health education centers, and private companies are providing a vast amount of initial training as well as continuing education. It is quite likely that many of your workforce development challenges would best be met through collaborative partnerships with these groups. One of the case studies in this book (Chapter Twelve) describes how hospitals in Northern California created an educational network for new workforce training and employee continuing education. These types of partnerships improve the quality of employee training and significantly decrease educational costs for individual organizations.

Building Tomorrow's Workforce

By working with local and regional education providers, health care organizations can ensure that potential employees are offered a variety of learning options. For example, community colleges offer many low-cost education programs and resources. By working closely with these colleges, the training and development department in your organization can influence the design of course offerings so that your workforce requirements are met. Some states have allocated funds for the development and maturation of regional consortia to rebuild health care workforces from the ground up.

Health care training professionals should also find out what career programs are offered by local colleges. These programs are designed to forge relationships between high school students and the world of work. There may be several opportunities for your health care organization to help groom the health care workforce of the future. Because most of the activity in workforce redesign and development is at the state level, Table 2.3 provides a listing of contacts and resources available in most states.

Continuing Education

Employees need access to a variety of continuing education programs: classroom training, on-line learning, journal articles, self-study systems, conferences, and so on. However, the health care organization no longer needs to lead the way in developing and presenting these programs. Never before have employees had so many different continuing education opportunities. On the Internet, for example, there are numerous programs that employees can complete in order to retain licensure and certification.

Training departments in health care organizations should assist employees in finding all the continuing education opportunities that exist and where appropriate partner with vendors to provide these opportunities in-house. The case study in Chapter Ten illustrates what can be accomplished when a health care system partners with a training vendor.

Table 2.3. Resources for Local and Regional Learning Partnerships.

Resource	Contact Information	Comments
Local workforce investment boards (LWIBs)	Contact: Local government Web address: www.usworkforce.org/wialaw.txt	This national Web address provides information regarding the Workforce Investment Act. For your state's information on how the proram is administered, log on to your state's Web site. LWIB may operate under the Regional Employment Board or through state Division of Employment and Training.
Local community colleges	Contact: Director of workforce education at your local community college	Community colleges offer workforce education and outreach programs in their communities. Available resources can be found through their Web site or by contacting the college.
Colleagues in Caring Project	Contact: Rebecca Rice Web address: www.aacn.nche.edu/CaringProject Phone: (202) 496-1093	This nursing workforce development collaborative is not active in all states. Check the Web site to access activity in your state.
Health care "corporate universities" University of Chicago Hospitals	Contact: Lisa Hunt Web address: www.uchospitals.edu/academy.html Phone: (773) 834-2668	This in-house model serves the learning needs of hospital employees and also provides access to multiple programs and conferences for hospital affiliates and external publics.
Healthstream University	Contact: Michael Pote, Senior Vice President Web address: www.health-stream.com Phone: (615) 301-3113	This model outsources many education and training programs to a health education vendor. This vendor offers a library of programs to clinical and management staff. Consultation services help organizations determine needs and focus their approach to employee education.
Mercy Medical Center Regional Education Center of Northern Iowa	Contact: Marge Wasicek Phone: (641) 422-7295	This model places the college within the integrated health delivery system with responsibility for all employee and customer training.

In addition, some health care organizations have formed "corporate universities" to support and sustain workforce development. Some are fully accredited universities that provide opportunities for students to earn a degree, while others are venues for sharing best practices (Meister, 1998). In general, corporate universities provide umbrella programs for all aspects of training using a variety of approaches. They can operate through a regional consortium of providers, outsource the training function, or provide all the training in-house. Table 2.3 provides information on three health care systems that are sponsoring corporate universities.

Creating partnerships with local and regional educational programs is an important fourth step in building a high-performance learning organization. Without such partnerships, it is unlikely that health care organizations can adequately meet current and future workforce needs.

Continuous Learning: A Key Strategic Objective

Health care delivery is growing more complex and diverse. At the same time, worker shortages are on the rise. These challenges require that health care organizations reinvent their learning systems. According to data collected by organizations such as the American Society for Training and Development (ASTD), one of the components that distinguish a leading-edge company is its commitment to and investment in learning. The business community increasingly recognizes that training the workforce is a win-win business strategy. However, it appears that the health care industry has yet to recognize that training is a key strategic planning element.

Compared to other industries, health care organizations spend a much smaller percentage of their payroll on training (McMurrer, Van Buren, and Woodwell, 2000). Continuous learning environments can play a pivotal role in ensuring that health care organizations meet strategic and performance goals. Effective training provides employees with the skills they need while addressing other problems such as staff turnover and workforce shortages.

It is imperative that health care leaders encourage new training approaches that link human resource and performance management with organizational goals. The model presented in this chapter illustrates one way this can be accomplished. Continuous learning environments create high-achieving organizations by fostering creativity rather than mediocrity and rewarding performance rather than mere existence. Through effective strategy and structure, organizations capture and share the experiences and knowledge of their workforce and establish measurable performance outputs that support critical business goals.

A continuous learning environment incorporates ongoing practices, integrating them into the organizational culture. Without an effective learning systems model, health care organizations will be ill equipped to meet the workforce demands of the twenty-first century.

References

American Society of Training and Development. "Investing in Workforce Training Improves Financial Success." Press release. Alexandria, Va.: American Society of Training and Development, Oct. 2000.

Bantleman, J. "Knowledge Management That Pays." *Evolve*, 2000, *1*(2), 28–31.

Herman, A. "Trends and Challenges for Work in the 21st Century." [http://www.dol.gov/dol/asp/public/future work/executivesum.htm] Nov. 2000.

Kaye, B., and Evans, S. "Retention: Tag, You're It." *Training and Development*, 2000, *54*(4), 29–34.

McMurrer, D., Van Buren, M., and Woodwell, W. *The 2000 American Society of Training and Development (ASTD) State of the Industry Report*. Alexandria, Va.: American Society of Training and Development, 2000.

Meister, J. *Corporate Universities: Lessons on Building a World-Class Workforce*. New York: McGraw-Hill, 1998.

Muirio, A. "Cisco's Quick Study." *Fast Company*, 2000, *10*, 287–295.

Senge, P. *The Fifth Discipline: The Art and Practice of the Learning Organization*. New York. Doubleday, 1990.

Watson Wyatt Worldwide. "More Employers Using Non-Monetary Rewards to
    Attract and Retain Talent." [http://www.watsonwyatt.com/homepage/gi/
    new/press.asp?id=7557]. Dec. 2000.

· ·

3

The Learning Transformation Process in a Health Care System

Diane Boynton, Donald C. Sibery

"A bold move!" "The end of 'business as usual.'" "Upsetting to the status quo." "Maybe just plain nuts!" These phrases come close to describing the early reactions to the cultural transformation learning agenda introduced to Central DuPage Health in early 1996. Central DuPage Health is a health care system located in the western suburbs of Chicago, with a workforce of four thousand employees. Since its founding in 1963 as a community-based, nonprofit, primary care hospital, the organization has developed into a diversified health care system. Central DuPage Hospital has grown in size and reputation, and the health care system has expanded to include a home health care agency, a primary care physician organization, five convenient care centers, a skilled nursing home, and a retirement community.

The case study in this chapter begins at a point in time when the organization was still adjusting to the experience of two distinct waves of reengineering, process redesign, and restructuring. In early 1996, local news coverage, the eyes and ears of the organization, and many hallway conversations were focused on potential merger negotiations that had been going on for nearly a year. In the midst of all this uncertainty, the board of directors was also conducting a search for a new chief executive officer. These were unsettling times in a workplace environment that had long been blessed by organizational vitality and growth and where a substantial number of longtime employees had spent most of their working years.

When the merger negotiations ultimately ended in spring 1996 in a decision not to merge, Donald C. Sibery assumed the CEO position. This was the starting point for the cultural transformation at Central DuPage Health. This revolution would eventually affect every aspect of the organization's leadership and staff development process.

An Unprecedented Investment in Learning

The learning investment begun in 1996 by Central DuPage Health has surpassed any previous education initiative. Four years into the process, more than three thousand individuals have enrolled in the classroom programs and educational retreats that make up Central DuPage Health's leadership development curriculum. Courses range from two-day training sessions to fifteen-day seminars offered over a period of ten to twelve months. Longer programs include substantial reading requirements, "homework," and coaching between sessions. The complete list of learning programs is presented in Table 3.1. Participants in the learning programs come from all corners of the health system—senior executives, frontline staff, new employees, physicians, employees in physician offices, and governing board members.

The educational process was begun with aggressive enrollment targets because of the belief that its ultimate effectiveness in supporting a cultural transformation would require a critical mass of learners and change champions. During the first eighteen months, three courses were offered: the Completion Series, the Transformational Leadership Program, and the Mastery Series. The health system budgeted more than twenty thousand hours for employees to attend these programs. By the end of the second year, the target of

Table 3.1. Leadership Training Programs Offered by
Central DuPage Health.

Course	Length	Participants
Completion Series	4 days	Senior executive, leadership staff
Transformational Leadership Program (TLP)	Varies, 6–8 days	Senior executive, leadership, and supervisory staff; physicians and physician office employees
Mastery Series	Varies, 12–15 days	Senior executive, management staff, physicians, board members
System Leader Program	4 days	Management staff, physicians
Winning at Work	2 days	All staff, all new employees, physician office staff
Trainer/Leader/Coach	12 days	Graduates of TLP or Mastery Series, through application process
Advanced Coaching Forum	12 days	Graduates of TLP or Mastery Series, through application process
Apprentice Program	2 days, with "practice" afterward	Graduates of TLP, Mastery Series, or Willing at Work, through application process
Reawakening the Spirit of Medicine	Varies	Physicians
Feminine Spirit Conversations	2 days	All women in the health care system
Breakthrough Project Training	Varies	Breakthrough project leaders and team members
Spirit of Service	3–4 days	Designated groups and inter-disciplinary teams

having two thousand individuals enrolled in the full curriculum of leadership and staff development programs was met. Most important, however, by the end of the fourth year, evidence of significant shifts and positive results for the organization was clearly emerging, including the following:

• Central DuPage Hospital's primary market share increased from 54.2 percent during the first two quarters of 1998 to 57.9 percent for the same period in 2000. (Secondary market share increased from 10.6 to 10.9 percent.) These changes occurred after a number of years of relatively flat results, and in a marketplace of this size, a 1 percent shift is considered sizable.

• The weighted average of mean scores for six key questions in the cultural transformation survey has continued to trend upward. It increased from 3.30 to 3.53 (on a 4.0 scale) from September 1997 to July 2000.

• Very favorable results of a Parkside Medical Staff survey (July 2000, with a response rate of 55.5 percent) included scores for overall composite quality and four of the subscales, which were two standard deviations above the mean.

In the early years of the new learning agenda, the availability and intense presence of experienced external consultants and facilitators was critical to the process. To meet this need, consultants from the Clarion Group (Seattle, Washington) were engaged to design and teach the original programs. These people worked onsite and were an important presence in the organization during the first year. Given the scope of this education process, the attention of the organization also had to be directed at strategies that would reinforce people's classroom experiences.

The learning transformation process at Central DuPage Health was much more than tools and techniques. A simple discussion of the steps taken to develop the training courses could not adequately address the underlying philosophies and strategies that were so critical to the success of the process. Other authors in this book describe the importance of a learning culture; it is our intent in this chapter to illustrate how health care executives can facilitate a culture change in their own organization. To meet this intent, the remainder of the chapter is presented in a dialogue format. This format allows readers to appreciate the actions as well as the thought processes that affected the development of the training program and the organization's transformation to a learning culture. The dialogue is between the authors of this chapter, Donald Sibery, CEO, and Diane Boynton, Director of Human Resource Development. These personal observations offer valuable insights into the distinct events, commitments, and strategies that helped Central DuPage Health maximize the organizational impact of the leadership and staff development process.

The CEO and the Trainer

Setting the Stage for Transformation

Boynton: Don, I recall the day of your first "public appearance" at a leadership team meeting in 1996. There was a definite buzz in the organization as word spread that you would be introduced to managers at the meeting. Many of us were presupposing what your first message to the organization might be. After being introduced at the meeting, you acknowledged the proud heritage at Central DuPage Health and stated your intent to continue this tradition. Then you shared your goal for initiating a process of cultural transformation. That got the attention of everyone in the room! Even though you faced multiple organizational priorities, why did you emphasize learning and cultural transformation so unequivocally in your first meeting with managers?

Sibery: Central DuPage Health was a destabilized organization at the time of my arrival as CEO. The organization had recently undergone dramatic reengineering and redesign. The health system was still suffering the frustration and embarrassment of a failed merger. The founding CEO of the organization was retiring, and people faced the realities of adapting to a new CEO. The organization was confronting some key issues: (1) people's willingness to embrace change as our friend and not an enemy, (2) the need to embrace physician leadership throughout the health system in order to tap into their profound leadership skills as we redesigned patient care services, and (3) the need to reduce our cost per unit of service. In my view, this set of challenges required more than the development of new management tools. People would actually need to shift their view of the world. Managers and staff were living in "scarcity" as a result of cost-cutting measures, and I needed them to be living in abundance as we went forward. People had become demoralized over a number of recent organizational failures. I needed them to move from a failure mode to one in which they were passionate about what we could accomplish in the future. This would mean that people would have to become vulnerable; not only connecting with their hearts, but actually bringing their hearts to work.

I also announced at the first meeting that it was my intention for the organization to be cost-effective in the marketplace—not by continuing to "hunker down" but by growing the organization. Through that growth, our per-unit cost of providing service would come down. I expected people to be more excited about growing the organization than merely just expanding cost-cutting tactics.

From my CEO perspective, although Central DuPage Health called itself a system, it was actually a number of different member organizations pretending to be a system. I believed that an organizational transformation would knock down barriers and provide a social lubricant that would allow people to interact with and listen to one another in a new way. Out of that interaction would come new partnership and possibilities.

Finally, at the front end of my tenure as CEO, I felt it important to give honor to the past but not let the past become a hitching post for the organization. Much of the organization's past was wonderful and memorable. However, the more recent past was tumultuous, stressful, and not exciting. If we were to move boldly into the future, those that viewed the past fondly could continue to honor it but also had to be willing to move in new and different directions. Those who viewed the past negatively needed to get beyond those attitudes. By speaking openly about their feelings and then putting the viewpoints squarely in the past, it would lessen the likelihood that these negative attitudes would be dragged into our future.

Boynton: Despite the recent past at Central DuPage Health and the mood you perceived upon taking the reins, why did you feel confident about initiating the cultural transformation process? Also, based on your own previous experiences in transformational learning, what barriers did you envision in our organization?

Sibery: I was confident that initiating the cultural transformation process would release a tremendous amount of energy and creativity within the organization. I was also confident that leadership would begin to emerge at all levels of the organization. Executives who believe that leadership resides at the top are actually living in scarcity rather than abundance. Leadership resides in everybody in the organization regardless of role, position, or education. I was convinced that as new leaders emerged at every level in the organization, they would take stands for change that would propel us forward.

At the same time, based on my previous experiences, I knew there would be major barriers to overcome as we unleashed transformational learning. As new leadership potential emerged throughout the organization, management could be threatened by new work practices. When employees speak honestly and straightforwardly and make very specific requests of their managers and attach timelines to those requests, this can make managers very uneasy. Managers are generally accustomed to being the decision makers and not used to being held accountable to the people they are leading. Any reprisals perpetrated on employees by managers for practicing new behaviors would kill the transformation process immediately. That is why we started the transformation work at the very top level of the organization, including the board of directors, physician leaders, and the system's executive team. The transformation work continued down through the management ranks during the first year and a half before it was rolled out deeply and broadly in the organization.

The barriers that I saw were on several fronts. There was a possibility of a push back from management and the senior executives as they started their own personal transformation journey. The "inner work" that transformational learning requires can be very threatening and unsettling. A second barrier that I anticipated was that as people do inner work and look deep into their heart and soul, it can become a very spiritual journey, and that sometimes creates confusion and raises questions about whether this is a religion. There was some consternation regarding this spiritual journey within the medical community and the organization at large. Over time, this has subsided as people realized that transformation work is not a religion but rather a means for personal inquiry. This inquiry often discloses paradigms or views of the world that people didn't even realize they had. More important, the transformation work never requires people to change their point of view or their paradigms. It is about gaining personal awareness so that people are no longer controlled by a particular view given the current set of circumstances they are dealing with.

Boynton: From the beginning, you repeatedly communicated three distinct themes and commitments: world-class listening, partnership, and agility. These were also dominant themes in the series of conversations you hosted with the board and the physicians. Why did you choose these factors to engage and unify leaders and staff at Central DuPage Health?

Sibery: I believe that nothing happens in the absence of a relationship. If the organization needs to move with great agility, there has to be a relationship with key stakeholders that was never there before. I also firmly believe that most people go through life desperately asking to be heard and seldom having that experience. So the commitment to world-class listening was made because it is a prerequisite to being a world-class partner, and both are necessary to developing organizational agility. I am talking about a kind of listening that comes from a place deep in a person's heart—namely, listening to what people are committed to. Through the transformation work, people learn to listen for the commitment behind the words of other people. Disagreements are frequently the result of words that are spoken and the interpretations we give to them. When people can get beyond the words and compare what they are committed to, often common ground can be found. This provides a basis on which a relationship can be built and people can move forward.

Partnerships that people stay in until a win-win solution can be found are crucial to our success going forward. True partners, first and foremost, listen to each other. True partnerships result in both parties winning rather than one party being subservient to the other party's needs. Central DuPage Health had not been viewed as a good partner. The organization had the tendency to dominate relationships. If things didn't go our way, we took our ball and bat and went home. The organization had a lot of work to do with key stakeholders to prove to them that we were trustworthy as a partner, and the transformation journey was a means to that end.

A "No Turning Back" Intervention

Boynton: Once Central DuPage Health began the journey of cultural transformation, we realized there would be no turning back. The process was fundamentally intended to create a vision of how the future was going to be different for our organization and an awareness of specific skills, competencies, and organizational attributes that would contribute to success in that future. So creating cognitive dissonance and disturbing the status quo were not simply by-products of the process; they were consciously intended. Once having ventured into those waters, however, there is no saying, "Oops, we didn't mean it!"

Designing the educational process and the change strategies that build momentum for cultural transformation has brought unique challenges and contradictions, twists and turns at every stage. I sometimes think of it all in the words of the Grateful Dead as "a long, strange journey," filled with the unexpected; and from a trainer's perspective, it has also been a very exciting endeavor. The scope is broad, the audience is diverse, and the curriculum is challenging. The learning agenda differs on many levels from traditional leadership development programs:

• This is a leadership development process that was designed to include staff at every level and in every sector of the health care system. It is based on the premise that the future will require leadership at every level in the organization regardless of role or position.

• This is not a "seven-step" or a "ten-step" program. It's not about developing a new technique or following a clever model for developing new leadership skill sets. Participants are encouraged to look deeply into their assumptions, values, beliefs, communication styles, behaviors, and practices. These attitudes have developed over time and are not easily abandoned or changed. Initially, there is a strong focus on looking inward, on reflection. Integrating lessons learned in the classroom with day-to-day work is not something that necessarily happens immediately. People may be slow to exhibit the personal development and organizational accomplishments that they acquire during the learning process.

• The organizational transformation provides an environment that allows for and encourages people to use what they learn. The environment makes it safer for people to put into practice new behaviors that might have been viewed as risky in the past.

• The cultural transformation is not intended to fix everything that is broken. The fundamental context for learning is self-awareness, understanding personal leadership capabilities, and breaking through barriers (many of them self-imposed) that limit one's full leadership potential.

All of these elements make the transformation process a long journey. By embarking on this journey, the organization was making a long-term commitment.

Sibery: Albert Schweitzer (1960) said, "You first have to be the changes you want to see in the world." The transformational development program at Central DuPage Health is not about tools and techniques or about "doing." There is a lot of action that comes out of the transformation work, but it is generated as a result of people shifting who they are "being" in the world. In a sense, the curriculum does not include a series of homework assignments but rather a series of life assignments. One of the major challenges in an organization is that the people have achieved a certain amount of success in their lives in order to be doing what they are doing. They have developed strategies that help them win in life, and often they are hesitant to give up those winning strategies even if they don't work anymore. So it requires strong commitment of people throughout the organization to serve as mirrors for each other, to provide honest, straightforward feedback for people as to what is working and what is not working. I believe that kind of culture needs to start at the top, or it will never flourish throughout the organization.

Facilitating the Transition

Boynton: Because this is a long-term investment in learning and development, the organization needed to plan systematically for key transitions over time. A critical shift has been from a consultant-led process to one that is primarily facilitated, coordinated, and supported by internal resources. The strategy for making this shift involved training an initial team of thirty middle managers and senior leaders, through our Trainer/Leader/Coach program, to facilitate the leadership development programs. This initial team also included the physician who served as chief of the medical staff at the time. Later, the facilitator team was expanded and reenergized through the Apprentice Program. This program was open to participation of staff at all levels who had completed the foundational coursework and who had a personal desire and commitment to cultural transformation.

Enrollment in the original Trainer/Leader/Coach Program and the Apprentice Program was based on a personal application process, as well as the recommendation of peers and colleagues and the endorsement of direct managers. This application process ensured that enrollees had an authentic commitment and desire to participate in the transformation. The organization viewed the application process as an essential element in the learning culture. It is believed that teaching cannot be "assigned," nor is it simply the responsibility of the organization's training staff.

Sibery: It was very important to kick-start this journey by using the Clarion Consulting Group as external consultants. However, it has been Clarion's philosophy, and my own, that we should not become consultant-dependent, not only because of costs involved but also because independence allowed the organization greater flexibility and agility going forward. Because we are talking about shifting the culture of an organization and then maintaining it with staff turnover rates being what they are, we had a consistent ongoing need to orient new people to the culture. This could best be accomplished over time by using internal rather than external consultants.

It was also very important for the senior executive team to co-lead the process, primarily because there is a certain amount of learning that takes place when you are a student and a very different level of learning that takes place when you have to lead. If the transformational work and the new culture were to be irreversible, the organization needed senior executive champions. The learning that took place among the senior executives during the first wave of courses was fairly new, and the root system was not very deep. As the organization picked up speed or encountered stress, the senior executives (like all other human beings) might revert to their old habits. I strongly believe in the adage that practice makes permanent rather than the conventional theory that practice makes perfect. When the senior executives co-lead programs, the learning from their own personal journeys will become part of a permanent way of being.

One of the difficulties in transitioning from external consultants is that at times you feel like the trapeze artist that has let go of one bar without the confidence that the other bar will appear as the right time to hold on to. As the external consultants stepped back, it created opportunities for new leaders to step forward. Some of our finest transformation leaders are not executive or management people. Other leaders have taken a step for themselves, their colleagues, and the organization by co-leading the transformation work.

External resources are used now as a mirror—providing us with an opportunity to see what we might not realize as an organization. I strongly believe that there is always a role for external consultants and resources, but they should be used for more focused and strategic issues. Outsourcing every aspect of the leadership development and transformation learning to external resources would be detrimental to the change process.

Looking Ahead

Boynton: In addition to building our internal capacity to lead transformation programs, our emphasis is also shifting now from classroom learning and formal curricula to building learning into everyday work and developing specific organizational practices to reinforce and "lock in" learning. This is an exciting phase because it is calling on the creative energy and contribution of individuals and teams at all levels of the organization as a community of learners. The response, for example, to our on-line "What if . . ." Question of the Week, which evolved from a very simple idea, has been astounding. This is a simple, cost-effective strategy, coordinated by Human Resource Development, that each week focuses the attention of the organization on an intriguing, sometimes provocative question. The response to the "what if" questions, which may be suggested and posed by anyone in the organization, continues to surprise us. Although no one is required to respond to these e-mail inquiries, our human resource department "chat line" is filled each week with amazing comments, possibility-thinking, provocative insights, creative suggestions, and personal dreams and commitments of employees from everywhere in the organization. Examples of these questions are presented in Exhibit 3.1.

Leaders also host spontaneous "think tanks" to engage people from all over the organization in conversations. Invitations to

Exhibit 3.1. Some "What if . . ." Questions of the Week.

What if, like Pinocchio, our noses grew each time we said the politically correct, safe thing?

What if we stopped talking in absolutes for a week? No "It is . . . ," "We must . . . ," "The truth is . . . ." And what if "I'll think about it" and "Interesting" were not acceptable answers?

What if we were to provide each of our patients with a personalized plan for the day, like breakfast 7:00–7:30 A.M., lab draws at 8:00 A.M., physical therapy 11:30 A.M., M.D. rounds 3:15 P.M., and so on?

What if the walls could talk? In the cafeteria, elevators, patient rooms, administration, your office?

What if all meeting rooms were converted to "open space" with an observation deck and you could drop in on any meeting? Which meeting would you want to attend?

What if, at our yearly physical, our spiritual well-being was assessed along with blood pressure, weight, diet, and the rest? What spiritual exercises or "diet" would improve your well-being in the coming year?

What if we were all growing younger and wiser? What would you want to do and accomplish in your ripe, young childhood?

What if you had a magic wand and could make any service improvement a reality today? What would you make happen? Why would you choose that particular improvement?

participate in these discussions are posted on the walls of our conference rooms and in other high-traffic areas. All interested people are invited to come and brainstorm, invent, critique, and dialogue on a distinct issue, question, or initiative. Informal discussions such as this are helping us build a culture of listening, partnership, and leadership at all levels, agility, and innovation.

This is not to say that classroom education will eventually end. In fact, the opposite is true. There is a constant recognition that our curriculum needs updating with new content. And other educational programs are being developed to foster the fundamental concepts of leadership development and cultural transformation. Enrollment practices have also changed. We now try to provide the opportunity for work teams to learn together. This contributes to the overall effectiveness of the classroom experience in several ways. When staff from the same work group attend a program together, it helps people support and coach each other back on the job. When improvement project teams have the chance to go through leadership development programs together, the experience creates an effective climate for building relatedness, seeing breakthrough possibilities, and ultimately accomplishing the project goals and objectives.

New Challenges, New Strategies

Sibery: As Central DuPage Health moves into the future, there are several strategic imperatives that will require us to embrace true paradigm shifts. One involves the reengineering and redesign of the way we deliver patient care and integrate acute inpatient, ambulatory, and physician office care on the main campus of Central DuPage Hospital. To accomplish the goals for this project, people will have to let go of the old view of the hospital being the center of the health care universe. Rather, people will need to embrace the philosophy that everything we do—the structure, the processes, the environment, and the people—is centered on our patients and customers. Patient- or customer-centered care will require our health system to be a world-class listener and world-class partner. To achieve our vision of having the healthiest communities in the United States by the year 2007, Central DuPage Health will need to be a world-class partner with the business community, the medical community, county and local governments, health departments, and human service and United Way agencies. The future for Central DuPage Health will require new kinds of organizational thinking. If we hold on to the past, there are limited possibilities for the future. Like many health care organizations, we need people who are able to move briskly into the future with a beginner's mind.

Our health system also needs to maintain what I refer to as "on ramps" to the cultural "superhighway" that is emerging at Central DuPage Health. Every day, new employees join Central DuPage Health, and even though they have not been part of the journey over the last four years, they are crucial to our future success. Therefore, the organization must continue to provide easy, early access to the transformation learning opportunities.

Finally, let me say something about the importance of a culture of coaching. The kind of coaching that I am referring to is not the same as what an athletic coach does. Athletic coaches frequently demonstrate what they want their athletes to do. The kind of coaching that I am referring to involves standing up for the success of the person being coached without providing advice or telling the person what to do. In this capacity, the coach serves as a mirror, allowing the coached individuals to see how they are viewing the world and a particular situation in order to discover their own pathway to a breakthrough or success. People do not need this type of coaching for things they already know how to do. People need coaches when they are taking on a bigger game and bigger future than they know how to accomplish. I believe a culture of this kind of transformational coaching will allow Central DuPage Health to achieve breakthroughs and have the kinds of successes we need to serve our communities best in the future.

Lessons Learned and Closing Thoughts

Boynton: Nothing has been simple or "business as usual" during the cultural transformation and the requisite reinvention of leadership and staff development at Central DuPage Health. There was no road map or prescription. In fact, we've learned that holding firm to a process that appears to be relevant and integrated with the real work and strategic objectives of the organization can actually be a hindrance. Holding steadfast to a particular process can cause people to lose their ability to invent, innovate, "try lots of stuff," and then try again. Organizations that choose to undertake a similar transformation must view it as a long-term investment. Otherwise, short-term tactics, "one size fits all" approaches, and the influence of other pressing priorities will soon sidetrack the efforts.

Sibery: There are a number of issues that I see more clearly now than I did four years ago. Organizations, like people, have a tendency when they are under stress to revert to their default settings and strategies that appeared to work in the past. The CEO has to be a guardian of the culture and stay involved in the transformation work until he or she is convinced that it is irreversible within the organization. Irreversibility does not occur when the only people that are living or embracing the commitment to cultural transformation are at the executive and management levels of the organization. Cultural transformation flourishes when it is nurtured deeply and widely throughout the organization. Cultural transformation is the hardest work I ever do as CEO. Many leadership teams give up because it takes so much energy over a sustained period of time. Finally, I've learned that there is no one path for an organization, nor is there a "right" way to realize strategic goals. To be effective coaches for organizational transformation, leaders must focus more on how we want people to be in the organization and not merely on how they get to that point.

Looking back over the last few years, I believe that the transformation work at Central DuPage Health has allowed people to move from the past into the future. It has allowed people to embrace change, and for the members of the system executive team, it has shifted their view of the unique contribution that physicians and physician executives can bring to our industry. When we began, there were no physicians on our system executive team. Today, five physician executive leaders sit on the team and actively contribute their critical insight, perspective, and leadership. Finally, the transformation work has clearly generated new enthusiasm and passion within the organization.

Boynton: As people work in an organization, over time they form beliefs and practices, which can become quite deeply embedded, about what to do, how to do it, and how to act in the culture. The transformation at Central DuPage Health has caused people to shed some of this armor. We are examining assumptions, beliefs, and ingrained strategies to gain access to a wider range of choices and possibility. Today, I believe that the essence of our learning and our transformation work has been about blurring the hard lines we've drawn around our "expertise," what we "know," and what we take as hard "fact." In a climate of dramatic and continuous change, this "clearing" is essential. People in Central DuPage Health are freer to try new things, take on new challenges, and contribute from the heart. This has been a very strategic organizational investment— one well worth making!

Reference

Schweitzer, A. *The Philosophy of Civilization* (C. T. Campion, trans.). Old Tappan, N.J.: Macmillan, 1960.

Part II

. . . .

Training Issues

4

• •

Training Challenges in
Health Care Organizations

Connie E. Kuykendall, Sally Zuel

Staff training and education are key to the fulfillment of an organization's business strategy. The U.S. Department of Labor has
determined that for businesses to achieve modest projections of
growth, better education and more job experience are needed for
the American worker (Deavers, Lyons, and Hattiangadi, 1999). The
development of worker skills has become essential to the economy.
Education and work-related training by businesses currently account
for almost half of the education courses taken by adults (Pantazis,
1999). Typical leading-edge organizations spent about $2 million
on employee training in 1997. The total training expenditure per
employee was $1,956 for those organizations. Of the benchmark
firms reviewed in 1997, health care organizations had the highest
percentage of employees receiving training, although the expenditure per employee and the percentage of the payroll were the lowest (Bassi and Van Buren, 1999).

The capacity to enhance people skills for the achievement of organizational goals can be one of a hospital's most important and most
valuable assets. Training can also benefit employees by advancing their
careers and enabling them to grow as people. If health care organizations are to achieve strategic goals, employee training initiatives will
need greater oversight and support from health care leaders. Companies are recognizing that our economy is dependent on knowledge,

and so it is becoming more critical to invest in ongoing employee development. Management theorist W. Edwards Deming noted that "improvement is not a one-time effort. Management is obligated to improve continually" (Walton, 1986, p. 66). It takes everyone and all areas, especially the education department, to accomplish this goal.

With the constant technology changes in the health care environment and shortened lengths of hospital stays, employees need to feel proficient in caring for patients. A feeling of proficiency comes from knowing what is expected and knowing how to use the various technologies in caring for patients. Staff will not continue working in an environment where the organization does not provide the education they need to maintain proficiency. Businesses are recognizing that staff retraining is less expensive than taking on new hires and that on-the-job training is a significant morale booster for employees. It is also a good recruitment and retention tool to have continual education for employees (Caudron, 1999).

This chapter describes the issues that senior leaders should consider when evaluating the current level and focus of staff education in their organization. Often health care leaders are passively supportive of staff education but lack a basic understanding of what it takes to have an effective training program. The information in this chapter is intended to broaden the knowledge of senior leaders so that more informed decisions can be made during strategic planning and budgeting for education services.

Scope and Structure of Staff Education

Hospitals that have an education department must determine quite clearly the scope of that department's responsibilities. Will the education department be responsible for providing training to only the nursing and other clinical staff? Or will the department be responsible for employee education and training throughout the entire facility? The scope of the education department's responsibilities greatly affects departmental staffing and the skill level of people working in that department. Instructors must know how to adapt training content and materials to people with varying levels of education and skills. Learning methodologies and program length need to be adapted to the target audience.

Senior leaders must decide whether the responsibility for staff education will be localized in one department or decentralized. Some organizations choose to provide a centralized overall orientation supplemented by department-specific orientations. Will some of the staff education responsibilities be outsourced? Consideration must be given to the costs involved and whether externally provided programs meet staff needs.

Capabilities of Training Staff

To function effectively, training professionals must understand the issues that the organization faces. These issues should be the focal point of educational content and programming. Staff education should be designed to help the organization meet its strategic goals. For example, if a goal is to improve patient satisfaction, employee training should be offered in areas such as patients' rights, telephone skills, and privacy protection. Improving patient satisfaction may mean that staff members need to be taught the importance of focusing on patient needs and how to meet those needs.

Staff educators must be able to understand varying needs of the targeted audience. Issues such as the average age of employees, levels of education and experience, and typical learning styles must be taken into account when training programs are designed. Staff diversity and its influence on training effectiveness is another factor that must be kept in mind when educational programs are planned. If the organization has a large number of foreign-born staff, educators must be sensitive to potential communication problems. Employee values can differ among various cultural, ethnic, and religious groups. Training content and presentation should be modified to address these differences.

The staff preceptors used for employee orientation programs must have sufficient experience and training. Securing adequate preceptor support can be challenging during times of high staff turnover. It may be necessary to budget additional time for experienced preceptors; otherwise, new hires will not receive the training needed to perform adequately. Consistency is another factor to consider when new hires have a preceptor or mentor. Orientees become quickly frustrated when they are assigned several preceptors and are told something different by each one. It is also important to give consideration to matching up orientees with preceptors who appear to be compatible with regard to age and experience (Anderson, 1998). Longer orientation periods can also be important for recruitment and retention. One researcher found that a longer orientation period increased employee participation and decreased openings in difficult-to-staff clinical areas (Bozell, 2001). Of course, the orientation should be tailored to the individual, since all new hires come to the organization from a variety of backgrounds and with a variety of experience.

Critical Training Elements

"Training that runs like a business never settles for what worked in the past. It seeks to be effective in the future. Another hallmark of training that runs like a business is clarity of mission" (Van Adelsberg and Trolley, 1999, p. 58). Several concerns are critical to developing a successful staff education program. Health care leaders should be careful to take the following actions in connection with their organization's education program.

1. Conduct needs assessments.
2. Define training objectives.
3. Identify training content and media.
4. Account for individual differences.

5. Evaluate training.

6. Revise training as necessary.

Needs Assessments

It is essential that the organization identify employees' learning needs. National standards and regulatory agency criteria set out requirements for education and training. These must be taken into consideration when identifying learning needs. Exhibit 4.1 presents the mandatory annual education requirements for staff at Union Hospital in Terre Haute, Indiana. Learning needs can also be identified through analyses of patient incidents, patient satisfaction survey results, infection control data, and other relevant performance data. In one organization that we know of, two levels of training are developed. First a core curriculum is designed to train individuals in basic skills and core competencies. Next the organization conducts corporatewide learning needs assessments to identify training needs that have strategic impact.

Employees should also be given an opportunity to identify their own training needs. In most cases, it can be assumed the learners can determine their own needs or at least learning wishes (Williams, 1998). Many health care organizations have recognized the importance of assessing the learning needs of their staff so that appropriate training and education can be designed to fill them.

Training Objectives

The learning needs assessment provides the information needed to establish the objectives of the training programs. Each training program should have defined observable behaviors that trainees are expected to demonstrate after the instruction.

Training Content and Media

Content represents the knowledge or skill that the trainee must master to be able to meet the behavioral objectives. People who

Exhibit 4.1. Mandatory Education Requirements at Union Hospital.

Annual Mandatory Education Requirements for Clinical Staff	Annual Mandatory Education Requirements for Nonclinical Staff
Cardiopulmonary resuscitation (every two years)	Customer relations, attitudes, and confidentiality
Corporate compliance	Fire safety and general electrical safety
Infection control and occupational safety	Hazardous materials
Ergonomics	Radiation safety (at the director's discretion based on the department's responsibilities)
Fire safety	
General electrical safety	Emergency and disaster preparedness
Hazardous materials	Ergonomics
Emergency and disaster preparedness	Age-specific competencies (required for all employees who come into contact with patients)
Security	
Medical equipment (as applicable)	
Age-specific education for patients served	Infection control and occupational safety
Restraints (as applicable)	Patient abuse and patient rights (required for all clinical departments that provide care or services)
Advanced cardiac life support (where applicable)	
Sedation and analgesia (as applicable)	
Radiation safety (where applicable)	
Patient abuse and patient rights	

know the demands of the job should help in defining the training content. Professional standards of practice and accreditation requirements must also be taken into consideration when developing training content. Another approach to defining training content is a problem-oriented method—the content is based on mistakes people are making in using a skill. Corrective learning measures are taken to reduce the likelihood of future mistakes. It is not clear which teaching method is more effective. Much depends on the specific training needs, the makeup of the student group, and other factors. Chapter Five discusses various training media and the advantages and drawbacks of each method.

Health care organizations should employ a variety of teaching methods to meet the needs of various audiences. The availability of resources is of primary concern when education is provided. Budgetary concerns affect decisions on length of programming, availability of supplies and equipment, teaching methodologies, and instructor-to-participant ratios. The limitation of financial resources has stimulated the use of creative techniques for providing the education, including Web-based self-instruction. Partnerships for larger programs can be developed with local universities, professional organizations, and other health care facilities. Financial support could be obtained through various vendors and benevolent organizations. However, it is important to remember that regulatory agencies sometimes place limitations on outside donations.

Individual Differences

Depending on their age group, employees have differing values and learning styles. The newest people to enter the job market are Generation Xers and the Net Generation. Generation X is the name given to the group of individuals born between 1965 and 1981. Based on the way they were raised and the upheaval they witnessed in organizations, Generation Xers have a unique set of behaviors, attitudes, and work habits. They have been characterized as technically efficient, independent, self-reliant, entrepreneurial, and impatient (Reese, 1999). These individuals are good at collaboration and consensus building and are typically self-interested. Generation Xers will stay with an employer as long as the employer offers something of value. Employers need to offer training, development, and growth opportunities to entice and retain Xers. This means, according to Jim Rapp (2000), that Generation X individuals must be

Challenged with assignments that allow them to use their entrepreneurial skills

Offered maximum interaction with others through a team environment

Provided clear directions and rationales about decisions

Helped with identifying potential career paths

Provided rewards when goals are met

Given frequent feedback

Currently entering the workforce is the Net or Echo-Boom Generation—people born after 1977. They have been bombarded with information and are media savvy. They have grown up in the digital age and are comfortable with changes brought about by new technologies and e-commerce. Individuals from the Net Generation are very comfortable with the communication revolution that has transformed every aspect of the business enterprise. Evidence suggests that people from this generation will excel in an environment where they can provide input on how work is done and propose innovative and creative solutions to improve workflow. Another asset is their strong sense of accountability (Alch, 2000).

Meeting the needs of the adult learner, of any age, can be challenging. Health care professionals appreciate the importance of ongoing education, especially with the continual change in technology. Staff should be included in the selection of the most convenient times and locations for educational programs. It also is beneficial to offer such things as frequent free workshops, paid education days, and overlapping shifts to maximize learning. Chapter Six addresses the needs of adult learners and offers recommendations on how health care organizations can meet these needs in a variety of ways.

Evaluating Training

Outcomes data should be gathered to validate the effectiveness of the educational program. Competency can be the outcome of learning, assessment, development, and experience (Aucoin and Puetz, 1998). Follow-up evaluation and feedback are critical for ensuring that a new process is appropriately implemented and maintained. Competency, as a means of evaluating outcomes, can also be measured by having people actually perform specific procedures such as sedation and analgesia. Chapter Seven provides a model for measuring the impact of training on important aspects of organizational performance.

Revising Training

The evaluation of training provides information as to whether the instruction had its intended effect. Were the learning objectives met? Seldom do the data indicate that a program was a complete success or failure, given multiple criteria for evaluating the results. Rather, the data may indicate better understanding, retention, or application of specific course materials. Gaps or variations in knowledge or competencies resulting from the training may reflect needs to consider more training time, alternative instructional techniques, or more capable instructors.

Improving the Competitive Edge Through High-Quality Training

Staff must value the educational programming provided if they are to incorporate the essential elements into their practice. The development of staff promotes greater satisfaction, higher self-esteem, and stronger commitment. This provides a basis for the development of critical thinking skills. A satisfying and thorough orientation and ongoing educational offerings enhance retention. When individuals are transferred from one area to another, they should be given an orientation plan that includes an evaluation of outcomes and competency.

The educational programming and process will be continually in flux. Organizations must take learners' needs into consideration and meet those needs in the most efficient and effective way. A way must be found to meet these needs cost-effectively while achieving positive outcomes. Resource management is crucial. And in addition to individual needs, the needs of the system as a whole must be considered.

Training plays a key role in an organization's competitive edge. Education and retraining are an essential investment in people. Health care organizations cannot maintain high-quality patient care unless the employees are continually gaining the new knowledge and skills that are needed to master ever-changing technologies and meet practice standards. When individuals are taught the appropriate skills and use them in caring for patients, it is a win-win situation for all.

References

Alch, M. L. "Get Ready for the Net Generation." *Training and Development*, 2000, 54(2), 32–34.

Anderson, J. K. "Orientation with Style: Matching Teaching/Learning Style." *Journal for Nurses in Staff Development*, 1998, 14(4), 192–196.

Aucoin, J. W., and Puetz, B.E.J. "Program Planning: Solving the Problem." In K. J. Kelly-Thomas (ed.), *Clinical and Nursing Staff Development*. (2nd ed.) Philadelphia and New York: Lippincott-Raven, 1998.

Bassi, L. J., and Van Buren, M. E. "Sharpening the Leading Edge." *Training and Development*, 1999, 53(1), 23–33.

Bozell, J. "The Midas Touch." *Nurse Managers: R&R Report*. [http://www.nursingmanagement.com/content/nm/0011/nmrr11.html]. Jan. 4, 2001.

Caudron, S. "The Female Profession." *Training and Development*, 1999, 53(5), 55–59.

Deavers, K., Lyons, M., and Hattiangadi, A. *A Century of Progress, a Century of Change: The American Workplace, 1999*. Washington, D.C.: Employment Policy Foundation, 1999.

Pantazis, C. "Individual Training Accounts." *Training and Development*, 1999, 53(10), 53–55.

Rapp, J. "Managing Generation Xers: As Employees, as Customers." *Office Systems*, 2000, 16(8), 14–18.

Reese, S. "The New Wave of Generation X Workers." *Business and Health*, 1999, *17*(6), 19–23.

Van Adelsberg, D., and Trolley, E. A. "Running Training like a Business." *Training and Development*, 1999, *53*(10), 56–65.

Walton, M. *Deming Management Method*. New York: Putnam, 1986.

Williams, M. L. "Making the Most of Learning Needs Assessments." *Journal for Nurses in Staff Development*, 1998, *14*(3), 137–142.

5

. . . .

Selecting Appropriate Training Methods

Brenda I. Mygrant, Mary Carole McMann

The educational process in the United States has evolved from a teacher-centered to a learner-centered model. This shift has reshaped the paradigms that guide all educational endeavors, including training strategies. One of the most valuable aspects of the learner-centered approach is establishment of clear, concrete training objectives. These objectives are based on organizational goals and identified workforce training needs. A model for linking an organization's strategic goals with performance standards and educational priorities is described in Chapter Two. Once the organization has identified strategic training requirements, the next step is to explore alternative training formats.

This chapter is designed to broaden your understanding of various training options available to health care organizations. An honest effort has been made to explain the relative benefits and disadvantages of each option, including some discussion of cost. Four learning approaches are covered in this chapter:

Lecture and small group training

Self-learning with printed materials

Technology-assisted learning

Mentoring

They are summarized in Table 5.1.

Table 5.1. Summary of Training Options, Formats, and Costs.

Learning Approaches	Methodology	Benefits	Cost to Construct Drawbacks	Professionally[a]
Lecture and small group training	Lecture Small group Workshop	Can reach larger numbers of people Can have small to moderate active participation	If audiovisual enhancements used, equipment failures can occur High time involvement for preparation and participation	Initial lecture: $6,000 for faculty and room Maintenance: $100 Audiovisual enhancements extra
Self-learning with print material	Monograph Slide show or lecture On-line article	Can control what is read	Can be time-consuming	Faculty honoraria: $1,000 to $2,000; up to $8,000 per member for monograph Slide lecture: honoraria plus $5 per slide
Computer-based training	CD-ROM with video, interactive Virtual reality media Multimedia	Can be loaded to server for multiple access Enhances user time during slow periods and increases interaction by participant due to privacy	Can be expensive if not a subscription-based program for updates Overall start-up costs can be prohibitive (though they are decreasing)	CD-ROM audio alone: $45,000 to $55,000 CD-ROM with video, interactive: $55,000 to $65,000 Interactive video: $4,000 to $5,000 per minute developed

	Asynchronous qualities (not all have to be on-line at one time) Increases learner retention Increases safety in exploring potentially dangerous subjects without risk Decreases cost per learner and average time spent by up to 50 percent	Dependent on systems in place and lost workload
Mentoring	Instructional mentoring (self-enrolled or department-directed)	Blends coaching, precepting, mentoring Increases role satisfaction Increases communication from junior to senior levels	Can decrease productivity, depending on technological enhancements Can be seen as punitive Success is dependent on effective mentor-mentee relationship

[a]Cost data were compiled by the authors on the basis of currently prevailing charges.

It is important to remember that any training strategy is only as effective as the organizational climate and structure that support the process. An organization committed to continuous learning sets long-term educational goals and does not fall prey to short-term fixes.

Introduction to Training Alternatives

Some educational formats are better suited than others to help learners reach their educational goals. While lecturers can quickly provide specific information to large audiences, techniques that promote active learning by the participants are typically better for teaching problem-solving approaches (Barrows and Tamblyn, 1980).

People can use almost any educational format to meet the continuing education requirements of professional licensure and specialty certifications. However, the same cannot be said for learning needs such as how to provide patient care or solve organizational problems. Health care workers should have access to several types of training options to meet different learning needs. Because some instructional techniques are more successful than others for teaching various topics, it is important that the right format be used (Schön, 1990). As illustrated in Table 5.2, the learner's retention of information is greatly influenced by the learning format. The sequencing of instruction and education is also important. For example, education for clinical professionals is often arranged sequentially—observation, hands-on experience, and then analysis (Cervero, 1990).

The selection of training methods should begin with an understanding of the target population. The educational formats that work well for the professional health care worker may not be as effective for lesser skilled labor. The existing skills of the target population are an important factor in determining the best learning methods. Next, a clear set of educational objectives should be defined. Thought can then be given to the various training alternatives for achieving these objectives. The educational formats that

Table 5.2. Rates of Retention for Different Learning Methods
and Formats.

Learning Method or Format	Percentage of Material Retained by Learner
Read monographs	10
Listen to lectures (includes audiotape, audio CD-ROM)	20
Listen to a slide lecture	30
Watch a demonstration and listen to a lecture	50
Participate in an active discussion of concepts (panel, debate, focus group, computer interactive)	70
Practice a skill, teach others a skill (role playing, real or virtual environment, hands-on skill practice)	90

Note: Data compiled from Johnson and Johnson, 1991.

are eventually chosen will depend on a number of factors, including the background and preferences of the learners and organizational constraints such as costs and available resources. Is the
training department in your organization using a systematic process
for selecting training methods? At a minimum, the following two
questions should be asked:

What possible educational formats could be used to help people achieve the learning outcomes?

Which of these formats would be most appropriate considering
the target population and other factors?

An understanding of the wide range of training methods that are
available to health care organizations is needed to answer these
questions.

Lecture and Small Group Training

The lecture style of teaching encourages superficial learning and is
the least effective educational format. Lecture provides people with
core knowledge that is abstract and is acquired passively. Audience

members learn whatever catches their attention, and although they may be able to recall the material later, they are unlikely to change their practices on the basis of what they recall.

Lecturing need not be completely abandoned; however, the problems that it brings to the educational experience of the health care workforce should be well understood so that it can be supplemented with more effective teaching methods.

When you are designing lecture programs, these are some of the important learning concepts that need to be considered:

- People cannot transfer learning from one setting to another.

- People are not pitchers into which knowledge can be poured.

- People cannot learn as an automatic response to a stimulus; they must think things through rationally.

- People's personal ideas and constructs affect their ability to learn new material.

- People should not be taught knowledge and skills separately.

The ultimate goal of education is to prepare people to function effectively outside of the learning environment. Studies have shown that learners do not predictably or effectively transfer lecture-learned knowledge to everyday practice. A passive learning environment such as a lecture may inhibit the learners' capacity to apply critical thinking or problem-solving skills. The participants may be able to "produce the right answer" or repeat the correct terms, but no behavior changes result. This outcome is common when learning occurs in a sterile environment, devoid of outside influences and disconnected from the learners' daily realties. When passive learners confront a problem, they tend to revert to the way they've always done things rather than adopt newly learned practices. The context within which education occurs is critical to the learners' ability to transfer what is learned and apply it to new situations.

Cooperative Learning

Any learning activity in which the participant does more than merely listen to a lecture is considered active learning. When lecturers incorporate exercises and other audience participation options, they are using active learning techniques. Cooperative learning, a subset of active learning, is an activity in which learners participate in small groups to complete complex tasks, research projects, and presentations. The time needed to conduct cooperative learning exercises can vary significantly. Exhibit 5.1 describes some common exercises used in classroom and small group educational sessions. The exercises are listed in ascending order according to the amount of time that is needed to complete the activity.

Small group learning can result in improved knowledge for the participants when the facilitator is an expert and the participants come from a variety of backgrounds or professions. When learners in this setting read relevant literature in addition to engaging in the small group activities, key concepts are reinforced, and changes in practice result. A review of cooperative learning techniques found that this format helps participants develop critical skills and greater social interdependence (Slavin, 1996). Other reports show improvements in learner retention (Johnson and Johnson, 1989, 1991).

Small group learning, particularly lecture-based small group formats, may be more successful and more appropriate when participants have similar job responsibilities. For example, when the learners have the same professional background and all work in the same clinic or hospital unit, the topics covered in the learning experience can be focused on day-to-day practice concerns.

A limitation of lecture-based small group learning is the need to have people participating at set times. If people don't feel the topic is relevant to their job, attendance may suffer. The availability of an expert to speak on a particular topic can also be a limiting factor.

Exhibit 5.1. Common Learning Exercises for Classroom and Small Group Educational Sessions.

Classroom or Lecture Learning

Goal of exercises is to increase student participation without interrupting the overall educational flow, increasing preparation time requirements, or increasing instructor grading or review time.

One-minute paper: Smallest time requirement; provides short written feedback concerning student retention and understanding of material presented immediately prior.

Take-home message: Provides short written feedback concerning student understanding of a group of lectures or presentations that are related.

Journals (daily or weekly): Usually topic- or point-oriented; can require a great deal of reading and writing, depending on the overall objectives and requirement for research.

Postlecture question-and-answer session: May require the most time because questions continue until desired answer is obtained.

Small Group Learning

Goal of exercises is dependent on the amount of participation and learner-instructed learning to occur in the amount of time provided.

Role playing: Smallest time requirement; limited to number of characters required to make the information flow.

Panel discussion: Entire group can be included in discussion in some manner, with a set number of panelists; preparation time varies by topic.

Debate: Subject matter must lend itself to pro and con argument; requires outside resources and preparation time; point-oriented.

Focus groups: Requires the most time; involves multiple sessions, moving from smaller focus groups that learn portions of the material to the full group learning it all.

Sources: Johnson and Johnson, 1989, 1991; Faust and Paulson, 1998.

Self-Learning with Printed Materials

The health care workforce can access a variety of printed materials to learn new skills and knowledge. The learning objectives influence the types of printed media that people need to meet educational goals. For example, textbooks are useful for refreshing basic information or reviewing past practices, but textbook information is not likely to be as up-to-date as that in a professional journal. If the goal is to practice "good medicine," the practitioner needs to determine what is recommended in current literature. This learning activity would include a MedLine search on a particular topic and retrieval of the pertinent articles for review. The availability of resources directly affects the success, costs, and limitations of this learning method. MedLine is a database of over eleven million references and abstracts. It is part of the U.S. National Library of Medicine, which links libraries throughout the United States and the sole purpose of which is to provide timely, convenient access to biomedical and health care information resources. The National Library of Medicine also maintains PubMed and Internet Grateful Med, two completely free systems with which to search MedLine on the Internet.

Although resources available on the Internet may not be considered "printed material," the information serves much the same educational purpose. Digital text and graphics can be downloaded for subsequent viewing or local printing or viewed on-line during a browser session. Many professional journals have on-line access to previously published articles. These articles are accessible directly from the publisher's Web site. In addition, Internet keyword searches can turn up useful references (Sullivan, 2001).

An Internet search engine that consistently delivers relevant results is Google, Inc. (www.google.com). The simplicity of Google's home page makes the search engine easy and fast to use. Google is one of the few search engines that delivers relevant listings that aren't top-heavy with pages from law firms and other vendors seeking clients. Unlike many search engines, Google's search technology also indexes Adobe .pdf files, a format commonly used to post educational materials on the Web. To achieve maximum benefit from a search, the use of a metasearch engine may be desired. The Dogpile search interface (www.dogpile.com) takes a single-line query and processes it so that maximum benefit is achieved from the search. Unlike other metasearch tools, a custom search may be performed for images, audio/MP3, streaming media, and the Web. Dogpile search includes a Google search as one of its fifteen search engines. Individual sites such as Medscape (www.medscape.com) offer original electronically published articles that cover a wide array of topics. Medscape's on-line search allows users to find references in its own library and on other Internet sites. Medscape's search engine is more limited in scope than either Google or Dogpile.

Conventional textbooks, journal articles, scripted slide lecture kits, and other printed and digital text materials are often used in self-study situations, although by themselves they do not ensure that learners master a topic. This is because printed media are designed simply to present information, not to provide a systematic learning program. For example, the practitioner who reads several journal articles on a new surgical technique is likely to broaden this educational experience through discussions with colleagues and specialists. Peer interactions and small group learning experiences help the practitioner incorporate new knowledge and skills into everyday practices.

Technology-Assisted Learning

Technological advances have had a profound effect on education and will continue to influence learning in the upcoming years. Technology-assisted instruction falls into two categories: computer-assisted learning and Web-based learning.

Careful planning is a necessity if organizations are to reap the benefits of the many new learning technologies. Computer-assisted and Web-based training can provide training in areas that are subject to frequent or periodic change; however, start-up hardware and software costs can be significant. A primary benefit of technology-assisted training is the flexibility of the learning process (Total Training Solutions, 2001). Unlike classroom training, which must necessarily occur at a specific time and place, technology-assisted learning can occur at any time and in almost any place. This flexibility can lead to significant salary savings. When IBM transitioned from classroom education for workers to "just-in-time" education with technology-assisted training materials, salary costs were reduced by 40 percent in some departments (Sambataro, 2000).

How was this possible? The $200 million in internal training cost savings were related to costs associated with traditional training sessions and time away from work. IBM provided its more than six thousand partners with ten satellite channels of product information. Receivers could be installed at any location, and for $1,500 per year, users gained access to up-to-date product-specific news as well as partner-related announcements. A Web-based system was set up to supplement the satellite system. This Web-based system allowed information to be known about a customer base prior to sale, thus enhancing the sales structure and adding to the overall profit of the company on top of the noted savings in training (Sambataro, 2000).

Computer-Assisted Learning

Advancements in software programming languages and the introduction of read-write CD-ROMs have greatly expanded the availability of computer-assisted instruction. There are numerous off-the-shelf training programs for health care professionals. Some health care organizations are creating their own CD-ROM training tools that teach institution-specific information. For example, your organization could develop a computer-assisted lesson that teaches people how to comply with your protocol for evaluating a patient's pain level. Developing this type of training tool does require that the programmer have some expertise in instructional design.

Computer-based training materials are generally very structured and can include many multimedia elements (text, high-level graphics, illustrations, photographic images, animation, motion video, narration, sound). Supporting materials such as hardcopy text or video can be used to supplement the CD. Computer-based training materials are useful when the consistency of the educational content is important and learners want to be able to access the information at their convenience.

Some computer-assisted learning takes the form of instructional presentations. Generally, this format uses sequential slide shows and may incorporate various multimedia elements. The training is basically tutorial, with little or no learner interaction. These formats work well as a quick introduction to a topic; however, the learner's ability to translate knowledge into practice is greatly increased when the instruction is interactive. Examples, exercises, and scenario-based learning techniques reinforce the content of the tutorial and help the employee apply the knowledge in real-life situations. Retention of the information is also greatly improved when the training is interactive.

Just-in-time (JIT) learning incorporates Web and Internet applications, CD-ROMs, satellite channels, and videotapes. JIT learning is particularly useful in quickly changing or high-turnover environments where workers need to continually update their skills (Sambataro, 2000). Workers can train at their own pace, wherever and whenever they like. Use of on-line JIT training cuts time involved by letting users grab only the chunks of information they need, conveniently from their desk. When comparing costs across the board, one day of conventional classroom training typically costs $500 to $1200, while one day of electronic learning averages $100 to $500. Cost savings can thus be more appreciable if training is slated for slow periods or if users are encouraged to zero in on just the information they need to solve a problem, perform a specific task, or quickly update their skills.

Many formulas exist to assist in establishing an overall return on investment when comparing classroom to multimedia training. Such comparisons are not always beneficial for smaller companies when establishing an average hourly benefit cost; however, one can appreciate its impact when looking at the larger concepts presented here. Tables 5.3 and 5.4 present a simplified example of such a cost comparison.

Web-Based Learning

Free Web browser plug-ins, improvements in bandwidths, and advancing programming standards have accelerated the development of Web-based training options. Internet sites providing audio slide lecture and live video-style lectures are increasing in number. The best-known medical multimedia training application of the early Internet (mid-1990s) was the National Library of Medicine's Visible Human Project (Ackerman, 1999). This database of computer-dissected cadaver slices was available to the public for educational, research, and clinical purposes. Today, there are a large number of Internet sites offering multimedia educational opportunities on topics of interest to health care professionals and the general public. Web access technology has evolved considerably, and people can now browse the Web using a variety of hardware. It is no longer necessary to have a full-function computer to access the Web. This revolution is making it less costly for organizations to purchase Web access devices for workforce training. In addition, health care employees are more likely to have personal access to the Web outside of the work environment.

Many of the training programs available on the Web are similar to the multimedia products used in computer-assisted training. However, it can be more difficult to evaluate the accuracy of information presented by lesser-known vendors, and you cannot always be assured that sites are providing up-to-date educational materials. On-line training materials offered by universities, medical professional groups,

Table 5.3. Determining Returns on Learning Investment: Multimedia Versus Classroom Training.

Classroom Cost Factors	Multimedia Cost Factors
Number of employees requiring training during twelve-month period (N)	Savings = $N \times L \times W \times 60\%$ (See Table 5.4 for a detailed example.)
Length of training (number of days per session of training per year; L)	
Average hourly wage of attendees (W)	
Percentage of employees traveling to location (outside normal travel to work location)	Savings involves no repetitive travel expenses. Expenses may involve computer or Internet expenditure, durable material depreciation.
Average expenses of lodging per diem	
Average airfare	
Average trainer salary	Cost is dependent on multimedia development cost.
Number of trainers required	
Number of classes per year	Learning can occur at any time; thus staff replacement costs are reduced.
Percentage of trainers traveling to location	No cost.
Program development costs (usually calculated per hour)	Development versus purchase.
Shelf life of program (usually not more than 24 months)	24 months for a slide lecture, versus zero for a subscriber Internet based learning opportunity.

Note: These data depict gross concepts only and do not account for any loss of workload, replacement of lost workload providers, or hourly benefits.

Table 5.4. Detailed Comparison of Costs Using the First Three Factors in Table 5.3.

Factor	Classroom Costs	Multimedia Costs
Number of employees requiring training (N) = 50 Length of training (L) = 2	50 × 2 $30 = $3,000 per year in salary	50 × 2 × $30 = $3,000 per year × 60% = $1,800 saved
Average hourly wage (W) = $30 per hour	Cost of salary = $1,200	
Shelf life = 2 years	$3,000 ÷ 2 = $1,500 per year (provided no salary or employee number increases)	$1,200 ÷ 2 = $600 per year (provided no salary or employee number increases)

Note: These data depict gross concepts only and do not account for any loss of workload, replacement of lost workload providers, or hourly benefits.

and well-established vendors are less likely to have erroneous or out-dated information. If the educational materials are well designed and continually updated by the developers, Web-based training can provide learners with the most current information on rapidly changing topics. If your organization wants to have more current computer-assisted training materials, product updates must be purchased.

Web-based medical education training programs are particularly useful when the learner can have a "virtual" real-life experience. This Web-based style of training can provide both a didactic and an experiential or explorative educational experience. For example, while learning about the workings of the gastrointestinal (GI) tract, students can "become" a piece of food that is first swallowed and then traverses the environment of the GI tract. The use of lifelike computer images of working body parts allows more realistic training than cadavers do. In cadaver work, the human tissue is different in consistency and color, and there are no body fluids. Furthermore, cadavers are not a renewable training resource. Once the learning experience is completed, a new cadaver must be obtained for the next student's use. When body parts are presented in virtual digital form, a real-life experience can be simulated and even complications can be vividly presented to students, over and over again. The learning experience can be repeated by any number of students without the need to purchase new "body parts."

Some health care organizations are using an intranet for workforce learning purposes. The value of this approach is the same as that of the Internet, with the additional advantage of being able to broadcast training materials that are specific to the requirements of the organization. For example, on-line intranet self-learning materials can be used to teach people about new medications added to the hospital's formulary or to comply with the procedures for a particular patient care unit. Internal creation of intranet training materials unique to the organization can be very costly, especially when designing interactive multimedia programs. An alternative is for health care organizations to join forces with Web-based training vendors to develop and maintain the programs. Chapter Ten describes a Web-based workforce training collaboration between Catholic Healthcare West and MC Strategies, Inc.

Mentoring

Mentoring is the process by which an experienced person provides advice, support, and encouragement to a less experienced person. A mentor is a teacher or adviser who leads through guidance and example. Mentoring can be an effective learning strategy in health care organizations. By deliberately pairing a more skilled or experienced person with a less skilled or experienced one, the less skilled person can grow and develop specific work skills and competencies. The instructional mentor can be a peer or a superior who advises one or more employees on job-related activities such as how to perform technical tasks, how to prioritize tasks, office relationships and etiquette, and professional work habits.

Many health care organizations use mentoring during a new person's orientation to the organization. The task is to learn about the organization and successfully adapt to a new job. In other instances, a longtime employee may seek out a mentor to help expand learning for career advancement purposes. In either role, the instructional mentor helps the learner search out and try new solutions, solve related problems, and correct errors.

Mentoring may be developed as a formal program or by a more self-directed approach. Both involve establishing objectives, finding and implementing learning activities, giving feedback, and evaluating process as well as progress for both mentor and mentee (Phillips-Jones, 2001). Instructional mentoring is often used as a positive solution to some of the problems of traditional in-service or small lecture group formats used to disseminate process and procedures. Used in this manner, instructional mentoring provides ongoing instruction and assessment of specific skills or organizational strategies. Such follow-up and professional dialogue are essential in organizations where educational training and philosophy can vary widely or where there is significant and constant turnover in personnel. Use of Internet resources, intranets, and e-mail enhance the mentor's time availability and clinical productivity. Without the use of such time multipliers, instructional mentoring has been noted to decrease productivity comparable to preceptors or by as much as 25 percent (Green-Hernandez, Marino, and Sansoucie, 2001). Emerging research on mentoring shows a relationship between mentoring and overall promotions, professional growth, and tenure in academia (Association of American Medical Colleges, 1996). Early studies show a relationship between mentoring and numbers of publications in peer-reviewed journals, time spent in research, and career satisfaction, all considered outcome measurements (Levinson, Kaufman, Clark, and Tolle, 1991).

Making Informed Training Choices

The surge of interest in educational outcomes has brought focus to the three factors that influence performance: ability, motivation, and environment (Cheren, 1999). Health care organizations can use various educational formats to address the ability factors. The range of learning options has greatly expanded in the past ten years, making it more difficult to select the best formats for the health care workforce. Limitations on educational budgets require that training options be carefully examined and matched to the learning objectives of individuals. Health care leaders may not be the ones who make final decisions about educational formats, but leaders should certainly demand that a systematic planning process be used in selecting training strategies. With all the new and exciting training options available today, the enthusiasm of training directors may need to be tempered by the questions of a knowledgeable CEO. New technologies are making workforce training more efficient than traditional classroom-style education. Computer-assisted and Web-based learning tools offer the organization cost-efficient ways of delivering high-quality education to a wide range of employees. To help employees integrate learning with practice, technology-assisted training should be supplemented with small group discussions and mentoring programs.

Leaders play a key role in the other two factors that affect educational outcomes—motivation and environment. A clearly articulated vision that creates the motivational climate necessary for continuous learning is more important than which training tools are selected. Knowledge is health care's most important resource. Organizations that fail to nurture this resource will find it increasingly difficult to recruit and retain employees, and the quality of patient care will eventually decline.

References

Ackerman, M. J. "The Visible Human Project: A Resource for Education." *Academic Medicine,* 1999, 74(6), 667–670.

Association of American Medical Colleges. *Enhancing the Environment for Women in Academic Medicine: Resources and Pathways.* Washington, D.C.: Association of American Medical Colleges, 1996.

Barrows, H. S., and Tamblyn, R. *Problem-Based Learning: An Approach to Medical Education.* New York: Springer Verlag, 1980.

Cervero, R. M. "The Importance of Practical Knowledge and Implications for Continuing Education." *Journal of Continuing Education in the Health Professions*, 1990, *10*(1), 85–94.

Cheren, M. "CME as Coaching, CME Director as Coach." *Journal of Continuing Education in the Health Professions*, 1999, *19*(4), 250–251.

Faust, J., and Paulson, D. "Active Learning in the College Classroom." *Journal on Excellence in College Teaching*, 1998, 9(2), 3–24.

Green-Hernandez, C., Marino, M. A., and Sansoucie, D. A. "National Organization of Nurse Practitioner Faculties 26th Annual Meeting— Nursing Conference Summaries." [http://www.medscape.com/Medscape/ CNO/2000/NONPF/public/index-NONPF.html]. Mar. 2001.

Johnson, D., and Johnson, R. *Cooperation and Competition: Theory and Research.* Edina, Minn.: Interaction Book Co., 1989.

Johnson, D., and Johnson, R. *Cooperative Learning: Increasing College Faculty Instructional Productivity.* ASHE-ERIC Higher Education Report no. N4. Washington, D.C.: House on Higher Education, George Washington University, 1991.

Levinson, W., Kaufman, K., Clark, B., and Tolle, S. W. "Mentors and Role Models for Women in Academic Medicine." *Western Journal of Medicine,* 1991, *154,* 423–426.

Phillips-Jones, L. "Professional Coaching vs. Formal Mentoring." [http://www.mentoringgroup.com/ideas]. Feb. 2001.

Sambataro, M. "Just-in-Time Learning." *Computerworld News.* [http://www.computerworld.com/cwi/story/0,1199,NAV47_STO44312,00. html]. Apr. 3, 2000.

Schön, D. A. *Educating the Reflective Practitioner: Toward a New Design for Teaching and Learning in the Professions.* San Francisco: Jossey-Bass, 1990.

Slavin, R. W. "Research on Cooperative Learning and Achievement: What We Know, What We Need to Know." *Contemporary Educational Psychology,* 1996, *21*(1), 43–69.

Sullivan, D. "2000 Search Engine Watch Awards." [http://www.searchenginewatch.com/awards/index.html#specialty]. Mar. 2001.

Total Training Solutions. "The Value of Using Interactive PC-Based Multimedia Training." [http://www.ttstrain.com/docs/value.htm]. Mar. 2001.

6

· ·

Training the Adult Learner in Health Care Organizations

Donna J. Slovensky, Pamela E. Paustian

Health care organizations are expecting much of more employees. Staff members must function as experts in certain areas
and still maintain the skills of a competent generalist. Work
redesign, cross-training, and the ever-changing new technologies
are creating an overwhelming need for on-the-job and formal training. Training systems in this new environment are being used to
help in redesigning the workforce to meet contemporary realities.
Staff education is critical in today's health care environment. Organizations cannot afford mediocre training programs. However, a
training program, no matter how well designed and administered,
loses effectiveness if it does not meet the needs of those it is sup-
posed to serve. A critical element in workforce training is the recognition of the needs of adult learners. For the purposes of this
chapter, an adult is defined as a person over the age of twenty-five
who has work and family responsibilities. The education and training functions in health care organizations are targeted primarily to
adult learners, and yet often the needs of this population are overlooked in program design and deployment.

There are some commonly held beliefs about adult learners—
they take pleasure in learning; they are self-directed learners; they
require a unique learning process. These assumptions may be true
for many adults learners, but some people, particularly those
involved in mandatory job training programs, may not have any of

these characteristics. What can be said of adult learners is that they possess years of life and work experience and a broad base of knowledge. Educators can capitalize on these strengths to enrich the adult learning experience.

One of the programs in the academic division of the University of Alabama at Birmingham (UAB) is designed specifically to facilitate career progression. This baccalaureate curriculum prepares associate degree clinical health professionals to move into mid-level manager positions in health care organizations. The people who enroll in these courses are all adult learners, often with ten to fifteen years' experience in demanding health care jobs. Almost all are employed full time and attend classes at night after completing a work shift. In addition, job skill training programs are provided to local employers on a contract basis. The participants in these training programs are full-time adult workers who have responsibilities to jobs and families in addition to their learning requirements. Our years of experience in working with adult learners in these programs have taught us much about the needs and expectations of these types of students. This chapter describes what we have learned about the issues that need to be addressed when designing and implementing training programs for working adults in health care organizations.

Issues in Educating Working Adults

Under most circumstances, teaching adults is extremely rewarding for the experienced educator who uses a variety of collaborative instructional methods. However, even experienced teachers will benefit from a review of key issues associated with adult education and training. Described in this section are the issues related to previous learning experiences, technology, competing responsibilities, learning styles, and personal motivation.

Influence of Previous Learning Experiences

Many people are affected greatly by previous experiences associated with school or training programs, particularly negative experiences.

For example, a person whose poor speaking skills were criticized in a previous training program may be hesitant to speak in front of a group this time. Individuals who struggled with algebra in high school may believe they can't learn statistical process improvement tools. A person whose self-esteem or ego is at risk may not ask questions or participate in learning. It is important to provide adult learners with a "safe" environment where they can admit lack of knowledge, acknowledge fears, and express differing opinions.

Trainers who recognize an individual's hesitancy to perform certain activities or an apparent lack of confidence in approaching new skills development can help learners overcome their fears in several ways. For example, trainers can provide positive feedback when performance is good. Similarly, employers can reward good performance through incremental tuition reimbursement based on the grade received in the course (for example, 100 percent for excellent performance, 80 percent for average performance, 60 percent for below-average performance).

Adults may have extreme anxiety about their ability to perform well in a formal education setting. Due to perceptions of the effects of aging, older adults may feel they are "out of practice" and unable to compete with younger adults in learning situations. They may lack confidence in their ability to learn new and different information and job skills. Some adult learners may need assistance in developing good study skills to improve their performance levels. Adult learners can also have significant test anxiety, particularly if the test scores are used to determine job competency and continued employment. It may be important to include in training programs a discussion of study skills and test-taking skills. These discussions can decrease the anxiety of adult learners and significantly improve overall performance.

A strong start in the educational process is an important success factor for adult learners. The initial contact between the instructor and the participants is a key opportunity to set the stage for a positive, energized environment that facilitates learning. Some general guidelines that instructors can use to create a positive first impression are presented in Exhibit 6.1.

Influence of New Technologies

Technology has become a key instruction delivery medium in many health care organizations. It is important to remember that many adult learners have only experienced traditional classroom instruction—lecture, pen-and-paper note taking, and written testing. Computer-aided instruction, multimedia presentations, job simulations, "virtual" classrooms, and other recent technological advances can be quite challenging for adults inexperienced with these learning tools. Even those who were skilled learners using traditional classroom methods may have difficulty with current teaching technologies.

Inadequate computer skills hinder the success of the adult learner. Although many health care professionals use a computer in some manner to do their jobs, most are exposed to only a few applications—usually proprietary single-function programs. For example, nurses log on to the information system, access the screens necessary for their job, and enter and retrieve data within specified

Exhibit 6.1. Guidelines for Initial Interaction with Adult Learners.

- Arrive early to greet and visit with participants.

- Let the participants get to know something about you. Tell them your background and qualifications for conducting the training program. Describe your teaching style and goals.

- Get the participants involved. Find out what their learning goals are, and encourage them to share information based on their knowledge and experience.

- Provide very specific information about the course or program, including expected learning outcomes, testing methods, and performance requirements.

- Be enthusiastic about your program. If you can't be excited about it, neither can your students.

- Show your sense of humor and encourage laughter. Demonstrate that it is possible to have fun while learning.

constraints. Many health care professionals have had little or no formal training in basic computer functionality and operation. When computers are used in classes or as a testing tool, a person's inability to use the computer may hamper the learning or test-taking process.

In the UAB's computer skills training programs, older adults often tell us their goal is to "catch up with the kids" or to "learn to talk about computers" in work or social settings. When the computer is demystified through explanations of the function of individual components and how information is stored and processed, the adult learners are better able to view the computer as a tool they control. Once the fear of the unknown has been conquered, computer technology becomes an enabler to learning rather than a hindrance.

Competing Responsibilities

Countless demands are placed on the adult learner's time. Work and family responsibilities, personal interests and hobbies, community or professional activities, commuting time, and various other activities compete for a share of people's time. Some health care workers may hold more than one job; others are caretakers for children or elderly parents (or both). Learning to balance competing priorities is a huge challenge that must be resolved on an individual basis. For many adult learners, work and family responsibilities take priority over educational endeavors.

This attitude has been observed in the students in UAB job training programs. One of our client organizations requires that employees attend a minimum of eight out of ten training sessions in the program to earn a certificate of attendance and a modest monetary stipend. Although the training sessions are scheduled after work hours, very few participants attend all ten sessions, and quite a few don't make the eight-session minimum. The adult learners skip the training classes to attend their children's sports events, to participate in church functions, to baby-sit grandchildren, even to work overtime on their jobs. To increase participation in the sessions by adult learners, self-study training materials are made available.

The financial burden associated with formal education and training is another issue that health care workers face. Although many organizations pay for developmental training and education offered by outside groups, the employee might be required to pay the tuition up front and be reimbursed upon successful program completion. Some health care organizations require continued employment for a period of time following completion of in-house training programs or school tuition reimbursement. Workers who are anxious about their ability to meet the employment requirements or financial commitments may be hesitant to participate in training. Associated costs, such as child care, travel, and lost work time, may be deterrents for some adult learners.

Learning Style and Readiness

Adult learners generally prefer learning activities that are task- or problem-centered. This means that learning activities should simulate, as much as possible, the real problems encountered in the worker's job. When learning is task- or problem-centered, adults are more likely to use the newly acquired knowledge or skill when they return to their job responsibilities.

Many adult learners prefer self-directed training. An effective educational experience is one that empowers people to learn on their own. This can be done by engaging learners in small group discussions and by using problem-solving exercises and case studies. Demonstrations and practice exercises can be used to guide students through the learning process. With adult learners, it is critical to consider the process of learning in addition to the content of the training program. Achieving the desired learning process without sacrificing necessary content requires careful attention to program design and skillful facilitation in the teaching phase.

To keep adults actively engaged in the learning process requires using multiple teaching approaches, most of which should be collaborative or interactive. Educators must use a variety of teaching styles and techniques appropriate to the desired learning outcomes. Frequently employed teaching styles include expert, role model, facilitator, and delegator. Teaching techniques associated with each style and the key points describing the techniques are presented in Table 6.1.

Lecture is typically the least effective method for teaching adult learners. Although lecture cannot be totally eliminated from most training programs, it should be aggressively supplemented with note-taking outlines, visual aids, discussion and questioning, and other participatory techniques.

Personal Motivation

Adult learners are generally very pragmatic, and "just-in-time" learning is typical of working adults. They tend to be more enthusiastic about training and education when the content is relevant

Table 6.1. Popular Teaching Styles and Techniques.

Teaching Style	Teaching Techniques	Key Points
Expert	Lecture Guided discussion	Efficient, good for delivering large amounts of required information; teacher or trainer controls content and process; predominantly auditory
Role model	Demonstration Coaching	Effective for teaching attitudes and behaviors; appropriate for teaching skills and techniques; provides how-to model; very visual
Facilitator	Application Problem solving Role playing Simulation	Useful for teaching practical, real-world skills; builds analytical and problem-solving skills; trainer and students share control over learning
Delegator	Independent study Self-discovery	Requires more time than other methods; builds analytical and problem-solving skills; gives student control over learning

to their current job or personal interests. Training programs should be designed with clearly established and well-communicated outcome goals that have immediate value for the learner. The benefit of gaining new knowledge or skills must be greater than the cost to the learner in terms of time or money.

Adults can be highly motivated to learn new skills that will improve their job efficiency or effectiveness. Some of our most interesting class discussions occur when students describe how they plan to apply learned concepts and skills to specific situations in their jobs. On the contrary, adults will be resistant to program participation if the course content is perceived as irrelevant to their job or at a skill level below their current competency. For instance, one of UAB's client organizations provided outdated instructional objectives for a mandatory job-training program. The objectives were linked to a specific competency exam that employees knew was outdated. At the time, the exam was under revision; however, testing was to continue under the old guidelines until the revised exam became available. The adult learners rightly questioned the value of "learning useless information" and regularly pointed out that "we haven't done it that way in years." Class participants stayed highly focused on (and resentful about) their belief that they would "have to go through this again" when the new test was available. To minimize student resentment, we not only prepared the employees to pass the current exam but also provided instructional materials that reflected the knowledge that would be tested in the future.

In all industries, including health care, job requirements change continually, and people need to learn new skills. To paraphrase the Red Queen, workers must learn as fast as they can just to stay in the same job. Workers count on their employers to bear a large portion of the costs associated with training. Employees commonly expect training to occur during regular working hours. They also expect to have little or no personal out-of-pocket expenses. Employees who want to move into higher-level jobs in their organization may aggressively seek out training and development opportunities. In these instances, people are more willing to accept some personal and financial responsibility for education and training related to career progression. An employee whose goal is to leave the organization may choose to pay all education costs to avoid job retention requirements.

Unique Needs of the Adult Learner

Adult learners desire active participation in the learning process. They expect to partner with instructors and trainers in directing the learning experience. Educators who lack the experience or desire to foster collaborative learning environments will find it difficult to teach adults. It is important to understand the needs and expectations of adult learners so that effective training activities can be designed and implemented. In this section, we share what we've learned from working with adult learners in formal classrooms, professional and executive development programs, and employee training courses.

Learner Needs and Expectations

Adult learners have achieved some level of education, job performance, and social status. They want to be respected as competent individuals. Adults also hold certain beliefs, values, and opinions, some of which may be well established and central to their self-concept. They expect instructors to acknowledge their right to hold those opinions and beliefs. Most adults are willing to explore alternative beliefs and opinions, even when their own don't change following exploration. The adult learners' commitment to their existing values is very evident when we conduct training sessions on professional ethics. As instructors, we know we have earned the students' trust and created an open learning environment when discussions about controversial issues become energetic and participants can't wait to voice their opinions. To improve learner participation, instructors should adopt a facilitator role—serving as a participant-observer and directing discussions with guided questions and comments.

Adult learners want instructors to facilitate the learning process but not to control it. It is important that educators acknowledge the competing demands for the learner's time and attention. This will often require that the planned training agenda be modified periodically. Adult learners are usually assertive in letting the instructor know when they need more or less time spent on a subject or when a particular segment of the training is not meeting their needs. The teacher who is unable or unwilling to allow this type of training flexibility will achieve little success in training adults.

The instructor must communicate clearly how the educational program is relevant to the person's current job responsibilities or how it will be useful in the future. As mentioned previously, adults are "just-in-time" learners who expect immediate utility from new knowledge and skills. They also learn better when new learning is connected to existing knowledge. Putting the content of the training program in the context of job requirements, impending changes, or external regulations can be very helpful in establishing learner motivation. Conversely, adults can be quite resistant to learning if the trainer does not understand their jobs well enough to create this connection.

Adults expect that learning will be fun or at least pleasant. They prefer congenial instructors and trainers who use humor. Adults expect to have personal exchanges with each other and with the instructor as a group and individually. People are by nature social beings, and they learn best when their social needs are met. We have found team teaching to be quite effective for many of our adult education programs.

Developing Learning Skills

Many adults have experienced only traditional classroom learning environments. For this reason, some people may not have developed the skills needed for today's work environments. For example, adults may lack skills in verbal expression, critical thinking, and multidirectional and creative thinking. Communication skills are frequently named as one of the most important personal and job skills for all workers, yet poor communication is cited consistently as the cause of many interpersonal problems. Trainers can assist people who are uncomfortable speaking in public by using focused questions and comments to initiate and guide discussion. Another important skill for the adult learner is the ability to listen. Researchers suggest that learners absorb only 20 percent of the information presented to them orally. Educators can assist adult learners by providing them with listening skill tips, such as paraphrasing or restating information, asking questions to clarify difficult concepts, and making notes to organize thoughts. An example model for active listening is presented in Exhibit 6.2.

Thinking skills—the ways people organize and process information they receive—deserve attention as well. Learners need analytical, critical, and creative thinking capabilities. Adults may need to be taught how to build frameworks that show relationships or patterns in information so that they can form opinions and draw conclusions. Most adults have experience with viewing information from a variety of perspectives, but some may be relatively unskilled at considering the influence of personal culture and biases on their decision-making and learning processes. For example, when students in our ethics class are introduced to the theoretical foundations of

Exhibit 6.2. Active Listening Model.

1. Give full attention to the speaker; note body language, type of information presented (facts, opinions, feelings), and action required.

2. Acknowledge the information by a nod or comment; avoid negative body language.

3. Encourage more information by asking questions or else remaining silent.

4. Summarize the information and repeat it to the speaker.

5. Ask questions to gain additional information or collect missing information.

ethical behavior, many are surprised to learn that their beliefs and behavior "fit" with the theory. Others learn that they had never thought about certain issues beyond their initial opinion, which in most cases was based on parental or peer influence.

Adults also have developed extensive vocabularies and knowledge frameworks. Therefore, exploring new concepts or learning new information may be difficult at first as they try to make associations with previously acquired knowledge. The instructor can ask questions or make comments that stimulate the learner to make connections and organize information to synthesize the new with the old. For example, when we use correct computer terminology to describe components or functionality in our training programs, many of the participants struggle until we provide specific examples. At that point, we learn the self-applied terms or descriptors the person has been using in performing the task. Once the connection between their words and ours has been made, they are able to adopt the correct term and incorporate it into their knowledge framework.

Creativity and innovation are essential skills that workers in health care organizations need almost daily. When people are not open to new ideas and no one directs any energy at being creative, the organization can remain trapped in the status quo. Everyone has the potential to be creative. However, some people repress their creative abilities, consciously or unconsciously, due to peer pressure, fear of failure, pragmatism, or other inhibiting factors. This repression may prevent people from finding new ways to perform tasks, solve problems, or explore opportunities. Techniques such as brainstorming and other freewheeling, idea-generating tools can be useful to stimulate creative thinking.

For most of our years of formal education, we learned as individuals. Adults, particularly in workplace training, need to learn to be able to learn in groups. The abilities to participate in group discussions, perform effectively as a team member, and reach collaborative solutions are necessary precursors to group learning. Trainers must be clear about the expected learning outcomes and facilitate the learning process to ensure that all group members participate. Participants need to feel that the learning environment is non-threatening and that diversity of opinion is permitted. Learners may need to be taught to build on another person's ideas and comments in a manner that fosters continued discussion rather than stopping it. It is very important for participants to be respectful of one another and acknowledge that emotions and personal exchanges can influence participation in the learning process.

Perceiving Adult Learning Needs in a Time of Change

For the workforce as a whole, changes in job responsibilities are a fact of life. All occupations, whether in health care or general business, have experienced dramatic changes due to technology. Organizational expectations are evolving with new reporting relationships, policies and procedures, and performance expectations. We have no reason to expect anything in the immediate future other than similar or perhaps accelerated evolution in the workplace.

Continuing education and training for all types of health care workers is an inescapable reality. To maximize the benefits of job-related training programs, educators in health care organizations must acknowledge that the adult learner has unique needs. Training activities must be designed to meet these needs. Given the opportunity, adult learners can effectively partner with instructors to achieve desired training outcomes. The "school years" paradigm of the teacher-student relationship does not apply when adults assume the role of students.

Adult learners must understand the benefit of gaining new knowledge or skills, especially when personal sacrifices may be required during the training process. Job training must be perceived as relevant, timely, and valuable. Trainers must use a variety of teaching methods with adult learners, placing more emphasis on collaboration and interactive assignments and keeping lecture to a minimum. Adults often bring extensive knowledge and experience with them, and they expect to be treated as partners in new learning opportunities. Thoughtful consideration of the issues and constraints that busy adults face is also an important factor when developing an effective training program.

. . . .

7

Measuring the Organizational Impact
of Training Programs

Richard J. Wagner, Robert Weigand

E arlier chapters have described the importance of a continuous learning environment in health care organizations and how to achieve training goals. What has not yet been thoroughly addressed is a question that is likely to be on the minds of many chief executive officers: Are these training efforts really paying off? This chapter offers some advice on how to answer this important question in your own organization.

Training programs can be very costly, and like any business investment, they must be regularly evaluated to determine continued worth. Assessment information can be used to decide if individual initiatives should be maintained, what is needed to improve program effectiveness, and whether education and training efforts have had a positive effect on organizational performance.

An effective training evaluation method helps support the organization's culture of learning. It says to employees, "We believe that training plays a critical role in this organization, and we need to assess its impact." The measurement process can assist leaders as well as staff in judging the bottom-line effect of training. By establishing a database of training results information and connecting the data to the training function, everyone will have a better understanding of the full impact that education has on the organization.

Surprisingly, the actual results of training programs are not often well measured. Studies reveal that fewer than 10 percent of staff education programs are adequately evaluated (American Society for Training and Development, 2001). Despite the cost of training, the value of the experience is often not adequately assessed. For example, a training exercise that is conducted with the goal of improving patient care might be evaluated by asking participants if they liked the program.

There are several reasons why the effects of training programs are not routinely measured. Probably the single most frequent reason is time—proper evaluation of a training program can take a lot of time, and health care workers are already overburdened with other duties. Many managers don't see staff training as an investment. It is classified as an indirect overhead cost and as such doesn't warrant intense evaluation. Measuring the value of training programs can also be inhibited by the difficulties in linking individual behaviors to organizational results. Often managers simply don't know how to assess the value of training programs properly, and many of the models proposed for this purpose are very complex.

It's unlikely that you'll prove beyond all reasonable doubt that training has had a direct impact on the organization's financial bottom line. Nonetheless, without studying the effects of training, it is hard to justify continued expenditures. That's why evaluations must be conducted for all staff training programs.

Training Evaluation Methods

A model for training evaluation, first proposed by Donald Kirkpatrick in the 1960s, is still widely used today (Kirkpatrick, 1998). This model involves four levels of analysis—reaction, learning, behavior, results—that are used to judge the value of a training experience.

> Level 1—Reaction: How did the participants feel about the program? Measuring reactions is a type of "customer satisfaction" indicator.

Level 2—Learning: To what extent did participants change their attitudes, improve their knowledge, or increase their skills?

Level 3—Behavior: To what extent did the participants change their on-the-job behavior?

Level 4—Results: What were the final results of the training session? Results include such factors as increased sales, improved quantity of production, improved quality, reduced costs, reduction of accidents, reduction in turnover, and increased profits and return on investments.

Different types of measurement instruments are used in evaluating each level. Satisfaction questionnaires are commonly used to assess participants' "reaction" to a training program. Some questions used to measure reactions are

Was this program really worthwhile?

Do we need more programs like this one?

Will the material presented help you do your job better?

Did the instructor do a good job?

Was sufficient time allotted for the program?

Measures of staff reaction to training programs may be easy to obtain, but the information is not generally helpful for determining whether the program was worth the financial investment.

Measuring students' "learning" is done through some type of written or observational skills testing. Such tests are ideally administered both before and after the training program so that the extent of change can be determined. While these tests are helpful at evaluating the immediate outcome of a learning experience, the results do not offer any insight into how improvements in staff performance are affecting the organization's financial bottom line.

Staff "behavior" following a training session is more difficult to measure. Evaluation techniques include work behavior observations, comments from peers and supervisors, patient satisfaction surveys, and "self-report" questionnaires on which training participants rate their own behaviors. Changes in staff behavior can be an indicator of the dollar value of training if the new behaviors are known to affect the organization's financial health (for example, use of less costly treatment options or better documentation of information used for billing purposes).

Financial Valuation Models

When the CEO asks, "Did training improve the organization's financial bottom line?" it is difficult to come up with a clear answer. Numerical data must be gathered to evaluate the end result of training programs. Two common formulas used for calculating the financial value of an undertaking such as training are the return-on-investment (ROI) model and the utility analysis model (see Exhibit 7.1).

Although both of these financial valuation models are applicable to training programs, it is usually difficult to find the needed information to compute the results. For instance, when using the utility analysis model, one must speculate how long the training benefits will last (T) and assign some type of objective valuation for D_t (performance differences for trained and untrained staff) and SD_y (dollar value of untrained staff's performance). Financial valuation models rely on hard data, but quantitative results showing the direct benefits of training cannot be defined with certainty.

Linking Training to Organizational Results

After years of frustrated attempts at measuring the results of training using various models, we began looking for a more meaningful system. This search began with interviews of literally thousands of

Exhibit 7.1. Formulas Used to Calculate the Financial Valuation of an Undertaking.

Return-on-Investment Model

The return-on-investment (ROI) model is expressed by the formula

$$ROI = \text{return (benefits)} \div \text{cost}$$

Utility Analysis Model

The utility analysis model is expressed by the formula

$$\Delta U = (N \times T \times D_t \times SD_y) - (N \times C)$$

where $\Delta U =$ dollar value of improved performance (or change in utility)
   N = number of people trained
   T = length of time the benefits from training will last
   D_t = difference in performance between trained and untrained employees (in standard deviation units)
   $SD_y =$ dollar value of untrained group's performance (in standard deviation units)
   C = cost of training each person

managers in many different industries, including health care. It was discovered that training programs were often designed and conducted without a clear understanding of the specific goals of these programs and with no thought given to how these programs could be evaluated. It was only after the program was completed that the question of value came up, usually when someone asked, "Was the program really worth the investment we made in training?" Since specific goals were never established, any evaluation after the fact was difficult at best. It soon became apparent to us that this process should be reversed. Program goals should be defined at the outset, with the evaluation process focused on measuring goal attainment.

Three-Step Evaluation Model

After completing our research, we designed a simpler, more pragmatic approach for evaluating the value of training program. This three-step training evaluation model is illustrated in Table 7.1. During program development (or sometimes after the program has been used several times), the goals of the training program are defined. In step 1, the goals reflect the staff behaviors that are expected to change following participation in the training (for example, a training program on managing patients' pain should make our employees more aware of patient needs). In step 2, the organizational results that are expected to improve by changing these staff behaviors are identified (for example, if employees are more aware of patients' needs, one result will be that more patients will return to the facility for follow-up or future care). Finally, in step 3, the expected behavior changes are linked to results that are already being measured by someone in the organization (for example, if patient returns are already being tracked, then select this measure to evaluate the effect of the pain management training program).

To expand on this three-step model, staff trainees and managers at St. Luke's Hospital and Health Network in Bethlehem, Pennsylvania, were interviewed. They were asked to name the organizational results mostly likely to occur when a training program has been effective. Ten key measures of organizational results (for convenience we call them organizational consequences) were identified (continued on next page):

Table 7.1. Three-Step Training Evaluation Model.

Step	Action	Sources of Data
1	Determine the behavior changes that will result from training.	• Key organizational managers • Supervisors • Training staff
2	Determine the possible organizational results that will be improved because of these behavior changes.	• Previous trainees • Supervisors and employees • Training staff
3	Link the behavior changes to results that are already being measured.	• Organizational financial managers • Key staff managers

1. Increases in efficiency and teamwork would result in improved employee satisfaction and subsequent decreases in job turnover.

2. Increases in efficiency would result in reduction of waste and lower indirect expenses for the hospital (materials, utility bills, equipment, and so on).

3. Use of fewer employees would save payroll and benefits costs.

4. Training and development expenses would be reduced, and so would direct costs (through such things as increased productivity and reduced labor costs).

5. Increases in job responsibilities through delegation would improve employee career mobility, enhance employee job satisfaction, and save the organization money through better utilization of employee skills in performing a broader range of tasks.

6. Cross-training would increase employee job flexibility, which would make employees more valuable because they are able to perform tasks that were previously done only by specialists.

7. Employees would experience less stress and burnout and would work together better. This would result in lower costs for health care coverage, less lost time from work, and lower disability costs.

8. Effective staff training would increase the occupancy rates at the hospital.

9. Effective staff training would result in increased revenue because a high number of patients would return to the hospital if they were satisfied customers.

10. Effective staff training would result in more satisfied patients, who would in turn recommend our hospital to others, thus increasing revenue and improving market share.

No training program is expected to address all ten of these organizational consequences.

In steps 2 and 3 of the evaluation model, people identify which of the ten consequences might be used to measure the results of a specific training program. These steps describe the critical linkage needed: Which results should change after attendance at a specific training program, and which of these results is the organization already tracking? It is important to know if data are available to judge the organizational consequences of a training program. If data are unavailable, the training impact cannot be measured. For example, if a particular patient care training program is expected to increase patient referrals, we would need to have access to data on the number of patient referrals both before and after the training program is conducted.

After applying the three-step evaluation model to several different training programs, we learned what has proved to be the most successful way to use the process:

• Step 1 (identifying the staff behaviors that are expected to change following participation in the training program) is generally best done through collaboration between the manager and the training department. Managers know why they are sending employees to training, and the training department knows the specifics of the training being offered.

• Step 2 (determining what organizational results may be improved by changing these staff behaviors) can be done by a number of groups in the organization. It seems most effective for new programs (or when evaluating an old program for the first time) to allow a small group of experienced former trainees to develop this important link. After a program has been successfully evaluated, this step can often be done by managers or by the training department.

• Step 3 (linking the behavior changes to results that are already being measured by someone in the organization) is often best done at first by management, possibly in consultation with the financial experts in the organization. Quite often data are available that no one has ever thought to ask for. This newly discovered data might be the missing link that is needed for measuring training results.

The three-step training evaluation model is designed to be flexible so that it can be used in a variety of learning situations. The real-life case study described in Exhibit 7.2 illustrates how the three-step evaluation process has worked in a health care facility.

Final Analysis

Once the training program is conducted and data are gathered, a final analysis is done. Continuing with the case study described in Exhibit 7.2, let's look at what the final analysis of the communication skills training revealed. While the specifics of the authors' consultative work done at various health care organizations must remain confidential, some general data that we have gathered will be used to illustrate the financial impact of the communication skills training program. The questions that should be considered during the analysis phase and the people who can help answer these questions are listed in Table 7.2.

In the communication skills training program example, we had additional information that made the analysis of the value of the training program even more complete—namely, the ability to analyze data from a group that did not receive any training (called a control group). The control group allowed us to determine if any changes we identified resulted from the training and not from some other cause. When dealing with a training program in which groups attend periodically, there is a built-in series of control groups to use for comparison. For example, if group A goes through training in January and group B goes in March, you can compare group A (trained group) with group B (control group) from January to March.

Exhibit 7.2. Application of the Three-Step Training Evaluation Model in a Health Care Facility.

The CEO of an independent health care facility in a small town was concerned to find out if its scarce training dollars were being used effectively. The CEO and the training director tried to figure out just how to determine the answer. They were most interested in discerning the bottom-line impact of their training efforts, but not surprisingly, they found that all their reading and research had not really given them the answer they sought.

The evaluation process began with the decision to evaluate a recently developed training program titled Improving Supervisor Communication Skills. The program had been previously given to two groups of supervisors, and the only evaluation that had been done was a reaction questionnaire (which suggested that the supervisors "liked" the program). Our first step was to determine the specific behaviors the program was designed to change. In a meeting with several key managers, it was determined that "listening to the employees" was a critical behavior that training was designed to improve.

A meeting was next held with a group of five supervisors who had been through the training program to determine which organizational consequences they thought should improve after this training program. They listed several possible results, including employee satisfaction, voluntary turnover, and "voluntary absenteeism." We took that list to several key managers for their agreement, which we received.

All was now ready for step 3 (linking the behaviors to results that are already being measured by the organization). This was done in a meeting with several key managers, including the human resource director and the finance director. At this meeting, we learned that voluntary turnover had been tracked for years but that employee satisfaction and voluntary absenteeism were not tracked.

Now we had a specific goal for the training program that could be evaluated using data the organization already tracked, voluntary turnover. We had this information from both before and after training, so we were able to track the change that took place as a result of the training. (How we made use of the data is explained in the text.)

Table 7.2. Questions to Consider During the Analysis Phase.

Question	Sources of Answer
Do we have data for before and after the program?	• Organizational financial managers • Key staff managers
Do we have a control group we can use?	• Training staff • Supervisors
What is the cost of the training?	• Training staff • Supervisors • Organizational financial managers
What are the benefits of training?	• Organizational financial managers • Supervisors

After completing the communication skills training, it was found that voluntary turnover for the group that had attended decreased from 15 percent for the quarter prior to training to 5 percent in the quarter after training. The group of employees that had not attended training experienced a 3 percent increase in voluntary turnover in the same quarter. Both groups were medical departments, and the people had similar skills and experience. It seemed fairly certain that the training program had reduced voluntary turnover. The financial return-on-investment data are illustrated in Table 7.3.

The savings from this training program exceeded the costs by $6,000 for one quarter. It is likely that this benefit will continue into future quarters and increase the savings even more dramatically.

Although this case study is a general scenario, it does show how this type of evaluation can be done with basic data that are commonly available at no extra cost. Can training program evaluations help the health care CEO and managers determine if the programs are having a positive impact on the organization's bottom line? Does this three-step evaluation model really help answer this important question? The most we can say is this: sometimes it can and sometimes it can't, but it is always worth trying.

Table 7.3. Financial Return on Investment for a Communication Skills Training Program.

Actual cost of the training program	
Cost of the program	$3,500
Wages for trainees	$4,000
Total cost of training	$7,500
Estimated savings from the training program	
Savings in recruiting costs	$2,700
Savings in training costs	$3,300
Increased productivity	$7,500
Total savings from training	$13,500

Quantifying the Value of Training

Training programs offer a wealth of benefits to any organization; however, they are very expensive to design and conduct. A lot of resources are consumed in direct programming costs, and the loss of output for trainers and trainees can be expensive. In today's cost-conscious health care environment, it is no longer acceptable to expend large amounts of resources on training and then hope that the organization will realize sufficient revenue to cover expenses. Training should be held to the same revenue-generating standard as any other program.

To calculate the financial benefit of training programs adequately, health care managers must learn how to quantify the organizational value of education. This starts with recognizing the behaviors that are expected to change following employee participation in the training. Next, determine what is likely to improve if employees adopt these new behaviors. The list of ten organizational results that are affected by staff training programs can be used as a guide in selecting measures of success. Ideally, the training program effectiveness measures will not add any new data collection requirements because information about these organizational results are already being gathered. By linking the results measures with training program participation, the CEO and others can quickly see if the education was successful.

The three-step training evaluation model described in this chapter will not answer all the questions that CEOs and managers may ask. However, by avoiding complicated formulas and subjective measures of trainees' reactions and by linking training goals to organizational results, there is a greater chance that meaningful cost-benefit information will be produced.

References

American Society for Training and Development. *State of the Industry Report, 2001.* Washington, D.C.: American Society for Training and Development, 2001.

Kirkpatrick, D. L. *Evaluating Training Programs: The Four Levels.* (2nd ed.) San Francisco: Berrett-Koehler, 1998.

8

· ·

Making the Most of Your
Training Dollar

Patrice L. Spath

The health care industry is experiencing reinvention, downsizing, and close public and regulatory scrutiny. Everyone that works in health care is being asked to "do more with less." To achieve organizational goals in this environment, employee education is crucial. However, training of employees is rarely popular. Training budgets are often the first to suffer under fiscal constraints and cutbacks. Yet staff education and training programs are indispensable in redesigning health care organizations to meet contemporary realities. Staff education is so critical in today's health care environment and education budgets are so tight that training programs cannot afford to be mediocre. Programs must be monitored and scrutinized carefully to ensure that they are of the highest quality. To make the most of training dollars, health care organizations must have an effective workforce training program that provides for continuous program improvement, enhanced participant learning, and improved organizational performance.

The purpose of this chapter is to describe the components of the ideal learning system in a health care organization. The recommendations can be used to benchmark the structure and elements of the learning system in your facility. If you find components that are missing or inadequately addressed, identify ways that your workforce learning system can be improved.

Oversight and Leadership

A multidisciplinary advisory board of people representing various hospital departments should oversee the staff education program. This board is charged with establishing training priorities, setting policies, and evaluating program outcomes. Advisory board members provide alternative perspectives and professional linkages that can directly and indirectly support the education and training of staff. Ideally, the advisory board meets at least quarterly to respond to emerging issues. More frequent meetings may be needed during new program start-up or in times of significant change.

The education advisory board should have a diverse membership that reflects both clinical and nonclinical groups. The people chosen for membership should be able to articulate staff training needs and concerns for their group. While boards vary in size, ten to twelve members are usually adequate to ensure sufficient representation of all stakeholders. The director of education should serve on the board; however, it may be desirable to name another person as chair. The advisory board should have a set of formal operating procedures that establish the purpose, membership terms, and other elements necessary to assist board members in understanding their role.

Training Programs

The staff education program should have a clearly defined process for the development and review of the training curriculum. The advisory board or the staff education department may perform this function. Training curricula should be reviewed at least once a year to ensure continued relevance to the topic and the organization's strategic goals.

Facilitywide staff training program must be linked conceptually and organizationally to the training efforts conducted in individual departments. This connection provides continuity and an opportunity to use training resources more effectively. The goal should be to develop a seamless training system within and between departments.

Staff orientation and training programs, no matter how well designed and administered, lose effectiveness if they are not accessible to the customers. Classes must be scheduled with a sufficient number of offerings to allow participants to complete the program in a reasonable period of time. Multisite health care organizations should consider offering classes at several locations so that participants' travel time is minimized.

Administrative and Financial Support

Staff education programs need administrative and financial support to expand training activities and to take calculated risks that lead to program improvement. Without such stability, a "survival" mentality develops. This leads to diminished risk taking by staff educators, less credibility of the training efforts among employees, and a decreased ability to attract and retain staff.

Financial resources must be used efficiently to keep training costs per person to the lowest level possible without jeopardizing program quality. Program costs, including per-person costs, are a frequent training evaluation measure. However, per-person cost without consideration of program quality may lead to poorly designed or badly managed staff education programs.

Where possible, the organization's staff education program should be linked to and supported by educators and professional associations. Such linkage improves the visibility and credibility of internal training programs. Formal linkages can be established with local colleges or universities and professional groups (associations, societies, and the like). Informal linkages, through endorsements, can also be established with outside groups.

Recognize training participants' achievements. Following completion of a program, participants should receive certificates, pins, or plaques that identify them as graduates. These rewards are important for the connections they create among training participants and for the enduring impact of a program.

Administrative Control

Staff education programs should have sufficient administrative control to ensure program quality without stifling innovation and creativity. Administrative control allows staff educators and the advisory board to track activity and make changes as necessary.

The staff education program must have a record-keeping system that allows managers to ascertain the training status of employees. This record-keeping system should also provide information that allows the staff education department to plan program delivery and evaluate training success. A variety of programs, from self-developed databases to off-the-shelf programs, can be used. The best record-keeping systems allow program staff to generate reports for individuals, for managers, for external review groups, and for internal planning and evaluation purposes. The information system should also allow for the identification of nonparticipants or individuals who have not made adequate progress.

Administrative control of the staff education and training program includes policies and procedures regarding attendance, testing, training program selection and completion, confidentiality, timely participation, and delivery options. The education program should also have well-defined procedures for the selection, orientation, development, and evaluation of instructors. Instructors (including staff mentors) should be oriented to the education program through a formal process. It may be helpful if instructors participate in an annual retreat or some other explicit training development activity. Program participants should evaluate instructors and the evaluative data provided to them.

The staff education department should have a well-defined and properly executed process for the development and evaluation of the training curriculum. The process should ensure that curriculum content and materials are current, relevant, and of the highest quality. Don't simply rely on materials produced by outside contractors. The facility-based staff educators should be involved in curriculum development and review and in program materials evaluation (for such matters as currency, relevance, and readability and copy quality).

Program Evaluation

Participants' learning should be evaluated for each training program. Both program administrators and participants use the information to evaluate program effectiveness. Each training program must have defined learning outcomes or objectives against which both instructors and participants are evaluated. Class evaluations can feed into the needs assessment process to ensure that established learning outcomes meet participants' needs.

Program delivery quality should be a component of this evaluation. Ineffective training delivery methods can hinder the achievement of training goals. Adult learning theory emphasizes the importance of using a variety of techniques and methods, both to respond to individual learning differences and to increase the likelihood that new information will be integrated into the learner's day-to-day practices.

Training participants' learning should be evaluated through structured processes. The transfer or application of classroom learning to a work setting is critical in adult education. Content-based examinations and work-related projects can be key parts of this process. Examinations can vary in formality, with some taking the form of standard in-class tests and others assigned as take-home exercises. Observation of participants' on-the-job behaviors can also occur at some time after training is completed. This kind of evaluation is time-consuming but is perhaps the best indicator that the training program has achieved its purposes.

Ongoing Evaluation

Evaluation of participants is a part of overall staff development program evaluation. Program evaluation should lead to corrections and improvements that allow training programs to respond to the changing patient care environment. Education and training programs can be evaluated indirectly—by examining class materials and other documentation and program management—or directly, through evaluation of classes and instructors. In addition, cost-savings information can create a comprehensive evaluation profile.

Staff education and training programs should have a process for ongoing or regular evaluation of all training materials used in the organization as well as of the procedures that support training activities. These materials should be scrutinized on a continuing basis to ensure that they respond to current conditions and needs. The advisory board may assume this responsibility or delegate the task to the director of staff education.

Where possible, evaluate cost savings that resulted from training. Cost savings and return on investment (ROI) have become increasingly important tools in decision making. The complexities of staff education and training in health care organizations make ROI analysis a difficult endeavor, yet any data generated from such studies can be very powerful in program improvement and survival.

The Staff Education Challenge

If senior leaders of health care organizations are committed to shaping the future of patient care and ensuring optimal patient outcomes, then staff education and training must be directed to meet these challenges. In the current health care economic climate, staff education and training programs that fall short of expectations risk ineffectiveness or extinction. How many of the components for learning system excellence described in this chapter are found in your workforce training program? If some components are missing or less than adequate, what can be done to improve your program? To make the most of your training dollars, your staff education program must be adequately managed and monitored.

Part III

. . . .

Training Solutions

Case Studies

· ·

9

Nurse Scrub Training Program Decreases Surgery Costs

Christina Dempsey

Challenges
· ·

- Decreased staff flexibility and dwindling numbers of qualified scrub personnel for recruitment

- Budget constraints regarding staffing

- Mix of registered nurses and surgical technologists falling short of "best practices" benchmark

Solutions
· ·

- Teach registered nurses to be proficient surgical scrub personnel as well as circulators in the operating room.

- Hire additional surgical staff to meet "best practices" staffing benchmark.

- Develop a clinically strong surgical technician and registered nurse first assistant program.

- Solicit support and assistance of staff surgical technologists in developing training programs.

Results
· ·

- A more flexible operating room staffing model with the skill mix approaching the "best practices" benchmark of 60 percent registered nurses and 40 percent surgical technologists

- An overall reduction in cost per procedure

- Learners with basic competencies for scrubbing and circulating with no further orientation required

- A collegial and mutually respectful working relationship among operating room staff

St. John's Regional Health Center is a 866-bed Level I trauma center in southwestern Missouri. The surgery department contains twenty-six suites with an annual volume in fiscal year 2000 of 23,719 patients. In the 1980s, a decision was made to increase the use of surgical technologists (STs) in the operating room. This decision was influenced by the shortage of registered nurses (RNs) and the hospital's budget constraints. By 1996, the skill mix in the operating room at St. John's was 30 percent RNs and 70 percent STs. Although this workforce appeared to handle the volume of cases adequately, the skill mix was significantly different from other hospitals. A 1995 survey of U.S. hospitals conducted by AORN (the Association of Perioperative Registered Nurses) revealed that the skill mix in most surgery departments averaged 69 percent RNs and 31 percent STs (Patterson, 1995). About the same time that the AORN study findings were published, employee morale was becoming a problem in the surgery department at St. John's. Surgeons complained about scheduling difficulties and inadequate equipment, and staff expressed concerns about patient care quality and lack of decisive action on the part of management. Staff frustration with the long-standing nature of several of these unresolved issues culminated in an employee walkout in January 1997.

Despite what might appear to be unique circumstances at St. John's, the underlying problems are very similar to the issues all hospitals face. Workforce shortages and budget cutbacks require the development of innovative, quality-focused solutions.

The case study presented in this chapter illustrates the important role that staff education played in resolving some of the problems in the surgery department at St. John's. Increased flexibility, improved quality, and decreased costs in the operating room were then, and continue to be, the primary goals. After a great deal of hard work, several new programs have been implemented to address these goals. One of the initiatives, a training program for nurses to prepare them for work in the operating room, is detailed in this chapter. Regardless of the circumstances that influenced the development of the new staff education initiative at St. John's, the program has merit and validity for all institutions.

Employer's Role in Specialized Training

A registered nurse needs highly technical and specialized skills to work in the operating room. Many of these skills are not taught in nursing undergraduate training programs. As in many health care professions, the undergraduate educational curricula for nurses focus on general knowledge and skills that are intended as a foundation for future learning. For specialized patient care positions such as those in perioperative services, employers must either hire experienced workers or provide on-the-job training for people lacking the necessary skills. In recent years, it has become more difficult for hospitals to recruit experienced surgical nurses, and the burden of on-the-job training is taxing the budgets of many surgery departments.

In response to these challenges, operating rooms have increased the use of surgical technologists; however, many perioperative service managers have found that when the level of RN staffing drops below 60 percent, surgery-scheduling problems can occur (Fernsebner, 1996). If a surgery department seeks to maintain an ideal ratio of nurses and technicians in the operating room, hospitals must find innovative ways to train newly graduated and seasoned nurses lacking the necessary special skills. In 1997, the low nurse-to-technician ratio at St. John's was already causing surgery-scheduling difficulties and was thought to be a contributing factor to low staff morale. For these reasons, the decision was made to increase the use of RNs in the operating room—a decision that required the development of a formal training program for scrub nurses. The RNs working in the operating room at St. John's in 1997 were trained to perform circulating duties but did not have training in scrub duties. To illustrate the difference between the perioperative duties of a circulator and a scrub position, Table 9.1 lists the common jobs these people would perform during a laminectomy procedure.

Historically, surgical technicians at St. John's had performed virtually all scrub duties; however, recruitment of new technician graduates for these positions was becoming more difficult due to decreases in enrollments at local schools. By filling open scrub positions with registered nurses and cross-training current nurse circulators to perform scrub duties, our goal of raising the percentage of nurses in the operating room could be realized. There was no intent to downplay the many positive contributions of the surgical technologists. The decision was made to train registered nurses for scrub positions because of the shortage of qualified scrub personnel and our desire to adjust the skill mix in the operating room to be more in line with perioperative services in other hospitals.

Another consideration was the flexibility that could be brought to the operating room by using RNs in scrub positions. Surgical technologists have excellent technical skills but lack the extensive clinical training and experience that RNs bring to the surgical patient. A registered nurse with dual training in circulator and scrub duties could perform either job when necessary. This would greatly relieve some of the surgery scheduling and staffing difficulties that occur when employees are at lunch or during shift changes.

Using more RNs was also seen as a way to increase the role of the surgical technician. For example, by using an RN to scrub and an RN to circulate for a case, the surgical technician would be freed up for duties such as opening another surgery room, covering cases

Table 9.1. Common Circulator and Scrub Responsibilities During a
Laminectomy Procedure.

Stage of Procedure	Circulator Duties	Scrub Duties
Preoperative (holding area and setup)	• Check readiness of operating room • Conduct preoperative assessment of patient • Verify that X-rays are available	• Check case cart for completeness and add supplies as needed • Scrub
Intraoperative (before induction of anesthesia)	• Assist anesthesiologist	• Set up supplies and equipment for surgery
Intraoperative (after induction of anesthesia)	• Assist in patient positioning • Apply ground pad • Prep patient	• Assist surgeon with procedure (retracting, clamping, passing instruments and sutures, suctioning and irrigating, and other tasks)
Cut to close	• Support operating room team • Complete documentation • Complete equipment and supply counts	• Assist surgeon with procedure (retracting, clamping, passing instruments and sutures, suctioning and irrigating, and other tasks)
Close to out	• Assist with undraping of patient and application of dressings • Check bovie pad and turn patient • Assist with patient transport to postanesthesia care unit • Assist with cleanup of the room and ready room for next patient	• Break down instruments, assist with undraping, assist with application of dressings, take instruments to decontamination areas

during staff breaks, or assisting with cases requiring additional scrub personnel. This was felt to be a more cost-effective way to use the skills of the surgical technologist. By having a higher percentage of RNs in the operating room, the depth of knowledge of the perioperative staff could be expanded. This knowledge could then be tapped for other projects such as materials standardization and cost containment.

The proposed change in the operating room staffing mix was expected to decrease overall costs in the department. Thankfully, hospital administration was willing to gamble that this assertion would prove accurate. Continued leadership support was instrumental in making the RN scrub training program a reality.

The Training Development Process

The initial pilot program added five full-time equivalents (FTEs) to the surgery department budget. This included one instructor and four students that would be enrolled in the training program. The initiative began in early 1998. The first challenge was to find an instructor who would be well regarded for her abilities and viewpoints by both licensed and unlicensed personnel. A current employee of the surgery department was hired to fill the position of RN scrub program educator. This person had worked her way up the ranks, having been employed in the operating room at several institutions throughout her career as a surgical technologist, licensed practical nurse, and registered nurse. This talented person brought to the instructor position many years of operating room experience and an abundance of ideas for making the program successful.

The RN scrub program educator spent most of 1998 developing a training program that incorporated basic surgical technologist curriculum, nursing policies, and scrub position skills. Considerable input was obtained from department staff, including the surgical technicians. The training format included lectures as well as laboratory simulations and preceptored experiences.

The course was initially designed to meet the training requirements of experienced circulating nurses. The pilot RN scrub program at St. John's included a six-month program of intense theory and didactic review of anatomy, physiology, surgical instrumentation, and sterile practices. In addition, students worked side by side with surgical technologists in the operating room for clinical experience and training.

Eventually, the training program was expanded to fulfill the more extensive educational needs of new nurse graduates who lacked both circulating and scrub experience. To accommodate these training needs, an additional three months was added to the program to teach circulator responsibilities such as documentation, patient safety, skin preparation, positioning, and patient monitoring. The complete course syllabus for the current surgical scrub and circulator training program is presented in the Appendix at the end of this chapter.

The RN scrub educator was also responsible for obtaining textbooks, a classroom area, and the equipment necessary for the training program, including a surgical table, instrument sets, and other surgical supplies for the simulated operating room lab.

Candidate Selection

During the time the RN scrub program educator was developing the pilot training program, the surgery department hired five new graduate RNs. These nurses received the usual on-the-job training for circulators so that they would be ready to replace the four experienced nurses who would be enrolling in the RN scrub training program. For the pilot project, it was felt best to use staff already familiar with the operating room and circulator duties. These people would require less time than new graduates to become proficient scrub personnel.

The circulating nurses selected for the initial scrub training program were chosen by a panel consisting of the surgery director, the

RN scrub program educator, the hospital's staff development coordinator, a surgical technologist, and a member of the surgery department management team. All experienced circulating nurses were offered the opportunity to apply for the training program. Eight of the fifty or so eligible nurses submitted applications. The panel interviewed each applicant.

This applicant selection process was considered fair and consistent with the team approach that had been used in developing the training program. When all interviews were complete, the four candidates with the highest ratings by the panel were selected. These students were paid their regular hourly wage during the program and also received free books and training materials.

The people selected for the training program were asked to sign a letter of agreement stating that they would remain employed in the department for a period of one year following completion of the RN scrub program or reimburse the hospital for the cost of their replacement (see Exhibit 9.1).

Details of the Pilot Project

The first RN scrub training program began in January 1999. Each day lasted from 6:30 A.M. to 3:00 P.M. The first twelve weeks were spent in classroom lectures where students reviewed anatomy basics and learned about surgical instrumentation and how to care for patients in surgery. The students were not expected to work overtime in the operating room or take call even though the operating room was occasionally short-staffed. The operating room director and the educator agreed that it was important for the people in the program to be students, focusing all of their attention on the theories and learning requirements of the course. It required great restraint on the part of the operating room management staff not to rely on these people in times of staffing shortages. However, the restraint proved beneficial. Students were given the opportunity to

Exhibit 9.1. Letter of Agreement Signed by Students in the RN Scrub Program.

Dear _____ :

In follow-up to our previous conversations, this letter shall serve as a letter of agreement concerning your participation in the RN Scrub Program. In consideration of the expenses paid and training provided, you agree to remain employed at St. John's Regional Health Center in the capacity as a nurse in the Surgery Department upon your completion of the program. You also agree for a period of one year following your completion of the program that you will not in any manner directly or indirectly be employed as a scrub nurse with any healthcare provider doing business within a fifty (50)-mile air radius from St. John's Regional Health Center. In addition, you agree to repay St. John's Health System at your current base rate of pay for any hours, as a full-time employee, under the one-year commitment at any time that you terminate your employment before the one-year commitment is reached.

If you have any questions, please do not hesitate to contact me. Otherwise, please acknowledge and sign below and return a copy to me as soon as possible.

Thank you for your commitment to this program and to the patients we serve here at St. John's.

Sincerely,

Christina Dempsey, BSN, CNOR
Nursing Director—Surgery

Acknowledged and agreed to this _____ day of _____ , 2000.

Signature: _____

focus on their studies, and everyone in the operating room saw that management viewed the training project as very important.

Twelve weeks after the program began, the students "interned" in the sterile processing department. Here they spent a week learning how to decontaminate instruments, put instrument sets together, and prepare equipment for sterilization. They were taught sterilization techniques and requirements. These exercises not only helped familiarize the students with the various instruments and setups for different procedures but also allowed the students to develop a collegial relationship with the sterile process staff. Each group gained new insights into one another's role in providing for the care of the surgical patient. This was a valuable and lasting side benefit of the RN scrub program. After spending a week in the sterile processing department, students were brought into the operating room. The stress of being the first students in a new program, coupled with the fact that many staff members did not embrace the program, was uncomfortable for some of the students. Some staff members felt threatened by the nurses who they felt sure were taking jobs away from technologists. However, constant reassurance for the nurses and incorporation of the STs in the program from the start eventually eased some of these tensions.

The educator had selected certain surgical technologists to act as preceptors for the students. These selections were based on the educator's previous experiences with the technologists, their abilities, and their willingness to participate. The RN students rotated throughout the different specialties in an organized fashion, learning skills in basic competency cases such as laparoscopic cholecystectomy, appendectomy, knee arthroscopy, tonsillectomy, hysterectomy, and some vascular procedures. They were taught to set up the instruments, anticipate surgeon needs, and assist during surgery. One week of training was spent on the evening shift so that students could have experience with the trauma and emergency cases typical of this shift. The students spent the last week of their training functioning independently as the scrub nurse for select cases.

Training Results

Regardless of how many years the "scrub student" nurse had spent in the operating room as a circulator, after completing the training all of them remarked on how much more they understood about the role of the scrub nurse. They believed the scrub training they had received would also help them be better circulators in future cases. They felt better able to anticipate the needs of the scrub nurse because they had a good understanding of how surgical cases progress. Many surgeons expressed a high level of satisfaction with the RN scrub nurses who completed the pilot program. The surgeons remarked that the nurses' technical training was very good, and they also had a very good understanding of the clinical aspects of the patients' care.

The students in the pilot program completed the training after only four months, two months ahead of the original schedule. A graduation ceremony was held, and each graduate was given a plaque acknowledging course completion. The day after graduation, these nurses were immediately put to work in scrub positions throughout the operating room.

Cost Savings

The true test of the program's success was in validating the original assumption that a change in the operating room staffing mix would decrease overall costs. The addition of RN scrub personnel in 1999 allowed the operating room to be much more flexible in scheduling cases and providing staff coverage. This resulted in an increase in the volume of surgical cases with an actual decrease in person-hours per patient. The data in Table 9.2 illustrate the cost savings realized in the program's first two years.

Having nurses trained in both circulator and scrub responsibilities has made it easier to relieve staff for breaks throughout the day. This flexibility has allowed for a more seamless day that has resulted

Table 9.2. Surgical Volume, Person-Hours per Patient, and Total Expenses per Patient, 1997–2000.

	1997	1998	1999	2000
Volume (number of surgeries)	21,643	22,097	22,551	23,719
Person-hours per patient	16.47	16.43	16.14	15.11
Total expenses per patient	$839.49	$1,016.55	$961.24	$958.73

Source: St. John's Regional Health Center, Springfield, Missouri.

in higher surgical volumes in the same number of worked hours. Case time in 2000 was, on average, seven minutes faster than in 1997. The overall morale of the department has improved due to the success of the collaboratively designed RN scrub training program. Several multidisciplinary task groups are currently working on other surgery department performance improvement projects.

Training in the Future

To date, four RN scrub classes have been held, and only one of the sixteen graduates has resigned from the department (to pursue a career outside of health care). Two nurses from outlying sister hospitals have been trained as well. The skill mix in the surgery department at St. John's is now 50-50 (one RN for every ST). This transition has taken place by simple attrition. Each year, more RN positions are added to the budget to allow for a smooth transition to the desired skill mix of 60 percent RN and 40 percent ST.

The training model for the RN scrub program is being used in a first assistant training program for registered nurses and surgical technicians. These training programs have enabled the surgery department at St. John's to maintain adequate staff while other hospitals are struggling with staff shortages and the high cost of hiring agency personnel. More important, the training programs have allowed St. John's to ensure that staff are adequately trained and competent to perform duties in the highly technological and specialized area of surgery.

Surgery personnel that have completed the training programs are proud of the accomplishment. They are great ambassadors for the program, the surgery department, and the facility. The success of the training programs has opened the door to other innovative projects. In the coming year, new nurse graduates and nurses without operating room experience will be invited to apply for the RN scrub program. Discussions are under way with local nursing schools to offer an "internship" program at St. John's for new graduates with an interest in surgery. Linkages with nursing schools will benefit the graduates and also help ensure that the surgery department at St. John's has a pool of skilled nurses to fill open positions.

The first assistant training program is still in its infancy, but it is hoped that this program can eventually partner with a local university to offer a Registered Nurse First Assistant (RNFA) certificate.

The past four years have been challenging, emotional, and rewarding for people in the surgery department at St. John's Regional Health Center. Through the hard work of many individuals, effective teamwork, and mutual respect, it has been possible to increase the skill mix in the operating room while decreasing overall costs and increasing volume. Administrative support and collaboration throughout the planning, implementation, and evaluation phases of the training program were critical to its success. The surgery department education initiatives at St. John's have improved professionalism and staff morale and lowered costs. These are goals that every health care CEO would like to achieve.

References

Fernsebner, B. "Building a Staffing Plan Based on OR's Needs." In P. Patterson (ed.), *Competencies for Management of the Operating Room*. Santa Fe, N.Mex.: OR Manager, 1996.

Patterson, P. "Editorial." *OR Manager*, 1995, *11*(10), 10.

Appendix
Course Syllabus, Registered Nurse Surgical Scrub and Circulator Program, St. John's Regional Health Center

COURSE TITLE: Operating Room Technique of the Surgical Scrub Nurse

INSTRUCTOR: Donna Broge, RN

COURSE MATERIALS:
Atkinson and Fortunato, *Introduction to Operating Room Technique* (Mosby)
Smith and Stehn, *Basic Surgical Instrumentation* (Saunders)
Meeker and Rothrock, *Alexander's Care of the Patient in Surgery* (Mosby)

COURSE RATIONALE:
To instruct students about the various steps of surgical procedures and the needed instruments, equipment, and supplies and to allow students to practice their skills in surgery, beginning with simple cases and advancing to more complicated cases.

COURSE DESCRIPTION:
This course is designed to instruct the learner to identify the operative sequence for surgical procedures. Emphasis is placed on surgical anatomy, supplies, and equipment needed for each procedure and surgical sequence. Classroom study will include surgical asepsis, surgical instrumentation, and basic lab skills. Included areas of study will be general surgery, gastrointestinal surgery, gynecology, genitourinary, thoracic, orthopedics, plastic, vascular, ear, nose, and throat, and laser surgeries. Basic ophthalmic and cardiac surgery will also be touched on. Students will be assigned to cases in the operating room, where they will learn to become proficient in their skills. Sterile technique will be practiced.

COURSE OBJECTIVES:
When students successfully complete this course, they will be able to
1. Discuss surgical attire, scrub, gowning and gloving
2. Complete a surgical scrub (five minute and three minute)
3. Don sterile gloves using closed and open techniques
4. Don sterile gown correctly
5. Remove sterile gown and gloves correctly
6. Gown and glove others
7. Apply the principles of sterile technique by
   a. Opening sterile package to provide a sterile field
   b. Opening sterile package to hand to sterile person
   c. Pouring sterile solutions properly
   d. Filling an asepto syringe and handling properly

   e. Proper handling of the specimen
   f. Changing places with another scrubbed person
8. Explain the principles of disinfection, sterilization, and skin antisepsis
9. Classify surgical instruments according to usage
10. Identify surgical instruments by sight
11. Hand instruments and supplies properly
12. Load knife blades on handles using a clamp or needle holder and hand properly
13. Load needles on needle holders for right- and left-handed surgeons
14. Thread and load free and french-eye needles
15. Hand free ties and ties on a passer
16. Wrap supplies for sterilization
17. Clean the operating room
18. Transfer patients to and from the operating room table
19. Identify instruments and supplies for each type of case
20. Dispose of needles, syringes, and all sharps correctly
21. Maintain an orderly surgical field so that she or he can be efficient and quick in handling supplies and instruments
22. Remove sharp and heavy instruments from the operative field as soon as surgeon finishes with them in order to prevent injury to the patient
23. Use universal precaution standards to prevent contamination by bloodborne pathogens of team members, patient, and self
24. Practice strict sterile technique to prevent contamination
25. Watch for hazards that would affect the patient intraoperatively
26. Receive and properly identify any medications or solutions
27. Identify and preserve specimens received during surgery
28. Count with the circulating nurse all sponges, needles, blades, and instruments, as needed; counts are done prior to, during, and at the end of the surgery
29. Watch the progress of the surgery in order to anticipate the needs of the surgeon
30. Assist the surgeon by sponging, cutting suture, auctioning fluids, and retracting tissue
31. Prepare instruments and supplies for decontamination and resterilization at the end of procedures; assist in safe room cleanup using universal precautions
32. Assist the surgeon and OR team in the types of cases listed in content outline

AMERICANS WITH DISABILITIES ACT:
If you have special needs as addressed by the Americans with Disabilities Act and need special devices or other assistance, notify your course instructor

immediately. Reasonable efforts will be made to accommodate your special needs.

ABSENTEEISM AND TARDY POLICY:
Near-perfect attendance is required to complete the required number of cases. Each student will be allowed two excused absences. A tardy is considered to be up to 6 minutes; after 6 minutes, it becomes an absence, you are allowed up to three tardies.

CLASS AND CLINICAL HOURS:
Classroom hours will be from 7:00 A.M. to 3:30 P.M. Monday through Friday. Clinical hours will be from 6:30 A.M. to 3:00 P.M. on Monday, Tuesday, Thursday, and Friday. Wednesday will be spent in the classroom. All clinical hours missed must be made up during finals week.

ADDITIONAL INFORMATION:
Each student will need clean shoes, safety glasses, and a name tag. The clinical instructor has the authority to send the student home due to illness. Conservative dress and appropriate manner and speech are expected.

GRADING:
This is a two-component course. The classroom portion is based on the following scale:

93%–100%	A
85%–92%	B
75%–84%	C
Below 75%	Failing

The clinical component is on a pass-fail grading system. Both components of this course must be passed in order for the student to complete the course. Grading for the practicum component will be based on performance, ability to follow directions, efficiency, speed, and safe working practices while performing sterile techniques.

CASES EACH STUDENT WILL SCRUB

GENERAL:
Appendectomy
Breast biopsy or mastectomy
Laparoscopic cholecystectomy
Bowel resection

GYNECOLOGICAL:
D&C (both suction and regular)
Laparoscopy
Vaginal hysterectomy
Abdominal hysterectomy

CARDIOVASCULAR:
  Carotid endarterectomy
  Abdominal aortic aneurysm (AAA)
  Femoropopliteal bypass
  Thoracotomy

UROLOGICAL:
  Cystoscopy
  Nephrectomy
  Radical prostatectomy

ORTHOPEDIC:
  Total joint replacement (both hip and knee procedures)
  IM rods
  Arthroscopy (knee and shoulder)
  ORIF extremities
  Amputations

PLASTIC AND RECONSTRUCTIVE:
  Skin grafts
  Carpal tunnel surgery (both open and endoscopic)
  Flap reconstruction

EAR, NOSE, AND THROAT:
  Tracheotomy
  Radical neck surgery
  Bronchoscopy

NEUROSURGERY:
  Craniotomy (both tumors and subdurals)
  Burr holes
  VP shunts
  Laminectomy (both lumbar and cervical)

CLASSROOM AND LAB

Week 1   History of surgery, expected behaviors of operating room personnel, accountability, guidelines for patient safety, ethical issues and surgical conscience

Week 2   The OR teams (sterile, nonsterile), the patient and his or her needs, potential sources of injury to caregiver and patient

Week 3   Attire, surgical scrub, gowning and gloving, essentials of asepsis, application of principles of aseptic and sterile techniques, sterilization and disinfection

Week 4   Surgical instrumentation, handling of instruments, cleaning of
          instruments, specialized surgical equipment

Week 5   Surgical instrumentation

Week 6   Tour sterile processing department and work there putting sets
          together, wrapping, and working in decontamination

Week 7   Setting up a sterile field, positioning patients, draping,
          instrumentation, hemostasis and blood loss replacement

Week 8   Factors influencing healing and infection, surgical wounds, wound
          closure materials, death of patient in the operating room

Week 9   Wound closure materials, general surgery procedures, equipment
          and sterile setup, peripheral vascular surgery procedures,
          equipment and sterile setup

Week 10   Gynecologic and urologic surgery, equipment and sterile setup

Week 11   ENT, plastic and ophthalmic surgery, equipment and sterile setup

Week 12   Orthopedic and neurosurgery, equipment and sterile setup

CLINICAL SETTING

Weeks 13–14   General and plastic cases

Weeks 15–16   Gynecologic and ophthalmic cases

Weeks 17–18   Urologic and ENT cases

Weeks 19–20   Orthopedic cases

Weeks 21–22   Neurologic cases

Weeks 23–24   Peripheral vascular cases

Weeks 25–26   Choice of clinical setting, makeup and final exam

Source: St. John's Regional Health Center, Springfield, Missouri.

10

Web-Based Training Expands Coding Education in a Large Health Care System

Gloryanne Bryant, Claire R. Dixon-Lee

Challenges

- Lack of consistent access to coding information and learning in all health care system facilities

- Need for corporatewide ongoing coding educational program

- Budget constrains regarding systemwide training

Solutions

- Implement a Web-based coding training program that allows for round-the-clock access to education with the ease of "click and learn" methodologies.

- Use the Web-based training solution to improve consistency and continuity of learning content and training objectives.

- Design a cost-effective Web-based training and education program.

Results

- The health care system now has a college level–coding curriculum equal to 160 hours that cost less than what would have been spent on seminars and workshops with equal educational value.

- Coding staff in all facilities are allocated hours for monthly educational activities.

- Coding training is consistent among all facilities in the health care system.

- Experience in implementing Web-based training will be useful when other routine education is developed for other employees.

Delivering high-quality and consistent staff education across a large health system can be challenging. Catholic Healthcare West (CHW), a San Francisco–based health care organization, met this challenge with a Web-based training program. Catholic Healthcare West consists of forty-seven hospitals and seven medical practice groups in California, Arizona, and Nevada. CHW facilities annually care for more than three hundred thousand patients and employ approximately forty thousand people. CHW operates with a chief executive officer and a board, with four divisional presidents and chief financial officers.

In early 2000, CHW identified the need for systemwide staff education on clinical coding and related reimbursement issues. In the past, CHW had a disparate distribution of coding education. Each facility had an educational budget for coding, and staff would attend a wide range of seminars and workshops. Some hospitals had independent consultants come on-site to provide education. None of the facilities was using the Internet as a training source or viewed Web-based training as a learning solution.

CHW's corporate director of coding and health information management compliance recognized the need for systemwide staff education on diagnosis and procedure coding. Several training-related issues were affecting coding processes at CHW facilities.

Billing procedures were becoming ever more dependent on timely and accurate coding of diagnoses and procedures. Increases in governmental scrutiny on health care had created a greater need for high-quality coding staff and assurances that coding practices were ethical and accurate. The U.S. Department of Health and Human Services (HHS) had made it very clear that health care providers needed to provide effective compliance-related training and education for all staff, especially in high-risk areas such as coding (Office of the Inspector General, 1998).

The Health Care Financing Administration's planned implementation of an outpatient prospective payment system (OPPS) in August 2000 was going to place an even greater burden on the health information management (HIM) services staff at CHW facilities. This burden was further complicated by the national shortage of qualified clinical coders. Prior to 2000, staff education for coders had been sporadic and inconsistent among the many CHW facilities. The training that did occur focused on the inpatient coding classification system. An extensive and ongoing education effort would be necessary if CHW facilities were to have a sufficient number of qualified clinical coders for both inpatient and outpatient services.

This case study describes the process used at CHW to select a systemwide coding training program for employees. The selection process included the establishment of clear goals and objectives for the program. Extensive research was conducted into the various training options currently available, which included printed materials, audiotapes, computer-based training, Web-based training, and on-site trainer-led workshops. Each training option was evaluated in terms of cost as well as ability to meet the learning needs of clinical coders in CHW facilities. After much study, CHW chose to implement a Web-based coding training program. This program was expected to be the most cost-efficient. It would help CHW achieve its goal of easily accessible, consistent, thorough, and up-to-date training for all coding staff. And the Web-based program could also be used to assess the capabilities of current clinical coding staff and support career development and training of new coders. This multiphase, systemwide program was begun in November 2000. Full implementation across the CHW system and in all affected departments was expected by the end of 2001.

Selecting the Training Method

CHW senior executives agreed that developing and sustaining a systemwide coding education program would be costly and time-consuming; especially since no formalized coding or reimbursement training programs were already in place. Although undertaking such an educational endeavor would be challenging, CHW senior executives agreed to the importance of the initiative. The goals and objectives of the coding education program are set forth in Exhibit 10.1.

Initiation of any training strategy starts with a clear understanding of the training goals and target population. The goal for the proposed coding education program was consistent with a guiding principle in the organization's compliance plan: to ensure that CHW employees have access to information that keeps them current with changing laws and regulatory requirements.

The internal education plan was to cover training of new or entry-level coders and updating of skills for existing coding staff. In addition, coders would need to be offered continuing education opportunities to assist them in maintaining coding certifications. Furthermore, staff involved in coding-related reimbursement activities would also need some training. The American Health Information Management Association (AHIMA) has published coding practice guidelines that address the core competencies of a certified coding specialist (see Prophet, 2000, pp. 73–75). Although coding certification is not an employment prerequisite at CHW, it was agreed that the AHIMA core coding competencies should be part of the education provided to the coding staff throughout the CHW system.

Exhibit 10.1. Goals and Objectives for Coding Training at
Catholic Healthcare West.

Catholic Healthcare West will provide consistent, high-quality coding education
and training to clinical coding staff and other personnel involved in the coding
aspects of reimbursement in order to

- Maintain compliance with the CHW Corporate Coding/HIM Compliance
  Plan
- Maintain case mix and accurate reimbursement levels across CHW facilities
- Assess, train, and retain highly qualified, credentialed coding staff
  throughout all CHW facilities
- Deliver educational programming that is economical, justifiable, and
  sustainable and has the potential to replicate training for other categories
  of CHW staff in the future
- Support individual, accessible coder continuing education at various
  skill levels
- Extend cost-effective coding training to other staff involved in the
  reimbursement process
- Demonstrate educational outreach in coding content to physician office
  personnel affiliated with CHW

Success of this program will contribute to increased coding accuracy, more
timely and accurate reimbursement, and better access to qualified clinical coders.

The target audience for the CHW coding skills assessment and
education initiative is varied and widely dispersed geographically.
This presented some unique learning challenges that had to be
addressed in the training design. To facilitate accurate and timely
coding and reimbursement, a number of hospital-based employees
needed to be included in the training initiative:

- Clinical coding staff in the HIM department
- Financial services and billing staff
- Patient registration and admitting staff
- Case managers
- Utilization review coordinators and select clinical and
  ancillary staff

In addition, the coding training initiative would involve staff working in CHW-affiliated physician practices and clinics.

The level of necessary instruction also varied among the target
audience for the coding training initiative. New hires and existing
staff responsible for assignment of diagnostic and procedure codes, as
well as people wishing to learn these skills, would have higher-
cognitive learning needs. Individualized training with directed self-
study, assignments, and mediated feedback would be required at this
level. Lower-cognitive learning would be provided for staff indirectly
involved in the coding aspects of reimbursement. Such learning could
be accomplished through lectures or self-study. Table 10.1 identifies
the basic content areas that would eventually be covered in the CHW
coding training initiative and the target populations for each topic.

An overriding objective of the CHW coding training initiative
was to provide instruction that is consistently delivered in all sites.
It was also agreed that education should be readily available to any
employee interested in or responsible for the assignment of diagnostic and procedure codes, as well as to more than four hundred
current CHW clinical coding staff in the acute care facilities.

Desirable Instructional Attributes

Once the goals, objectives, and target audiences for the coding
training initiative were clearly understood, a list of desirable attributes for the instructional method was developed. The ideal training method should meet the following requirements:

- It should be flexible.

- It should be available around the clock.

- It should allow for facility-based administrator
  monitoring and oversight.

- It should provide user-friendly report production.

- It should be easy to update.

Table 10.1. Topic Content Areas and Target Training Populations.

	Target Training Population		
Topic Content Area[a]	People wishing to learn coding skills	People with coding skills (new hires and existing staff)	People indirectly involved in coding and reimbursement
Reimbursement methodologies	•	•	•
Medical terminology	•	•	•
Legal, ethical, and compliance issues affecting reimbursement	•	•	•
Basic ICD-9-CM coding principles	•	•	•
Basic CPT-4 coding principles	•	•	•
Advanced ICD-9-CM coding principles	•	•	
Advanced CPT-4/HCPCS coding principles	•	•	
Ambulatory payment classifications	•	•	•
Recent changes in reimbursement practices or coding principles	•	•	
Physician office coding principles	•	•	•

[a] ICD-9-CM stands for International Classification of Diseases, 9th Revision, Clinical Modification; CPT-4 stands for the American Medical Association's Current Procedural Terminology; HCPCS stands for the U.S. Health Care Financing Administration's Common Procedure Coding System.

All of the currently available training options were explored and matched against these desirable elements. There are seven predominant methods for training large numbers of individuals in coding and compliance topics:

Small group classroom training

Seminar lectures

Audio or video teleconferencing

Video instruction

Custom-developed interactive multimedia training

Computer-based training

Web-based training

Let us examine the advantages and disadvantages of each.

Classroom Instruction

Classroom instruction can be excellent for team building and motivating individuals to action. The classroom also provides a good format for developing relationships and for practicing lessons and techniques learned by using activities such as role playing or problem solving. It is the best medium for delivering, discussing, and emphasizing ideas and concepts; however, self-directed learning is usually more effective for teaching technical material such as clinical coding. For health care compliance topics, an extensive number of issues and an immense amount of technical content and depth must be covered in training programs. The content often applies only to specialty groups with small numbers of individuals. The large number of topics and sometimes small numbers of individuals to whom the content may apply makes classroom delivery an unmanageable option for the coding and compliance training program at CHW facilities.

Seminars

Seminars are a good format for delivering instructional materials to a large group of people. Seminars can be used to deliver, discuss, and emphasize ideas and concepts. However, seminars are a less effective method for learning technical material. Other disadvantages include the need to schedule seminars on a particular date, the expense of student travel (if required), and the generic nature of the content necessitated by the large and often diverse audience. Since the coding and compliance training program at CHW would be provided to a small, specialized group of employers, seminars were viewed as an expensive training alternative with limited application.

Audio or Video Teleconferencing

Teleconferences can provide potentially high-quality instructors and learning content that might not otherwise be available for large audiences. Teleconferences are also an excellent means for emphasizing the importance of a subject or motivating the learner to action. However, teleconferencing has many of the same disadvantages as seminars: scheduling difficulties (coordination of staff schedules, classroom scheduling, facilitator preparation, site equipment), questionable suitability for technical subject matter, and the generic nature of the content. In addition, the teleconferencing technology itself can be problematic; the audio or video may be of poor quality. Self-directed learning is generally more effective for learning technical topics such as coding. When teaching coding concepts and requirements, an extensive amount of material must be covered, and this could greatly raise the cost of teleconference-based training. Teleconferencing is more cost-effective for narrowly focused topics that have a broad audience, such as new regulations or guidelines.

Video Instruction

Videos offer a flexible option for training: they are readily available, can be viewed on demand, and can be viewed at or near the workstation. Many learners prefer visual training. The most significant drawbacks of videos are that the content is fixed and is often quickly outdated, especially for clinical coding topics. Also, videos are not interactive unless used in a classroom setting with a facilitator. Often coding staff need interactive training to foster analytical and problem-solving skills.

Custom-Developed Interactive Multimedia Training

Internal development of interactive multimedia training (IMT) is an option for organizations with large information systems and instructional design capabilities. The advantages of internally developed training materials include the ability to tailor all content specifically to the institution and to manage in-house all required updates and priorities for new development. All the numerous advantages of self-directed learning and use of IMT applications can accrue to the learner and the organization with this approach. The major difficulty of IMT is in developing the internal capability to write and produce the hundreds of hours of technical material necessary to meet the diverse needs of learners and then keep all the material updated. In addition, updating the functionality of the software can also be a major challenge.

Computer-Based Training

Computer-based training (CBT) platforms are available to assist organizations with large information systems and instructional design capabilities that wish to develop their own content. The development tools for converting written materials to CBT are readily available and are becoming easier to use. The advantages and disadvantages of internally developed CBT are very similar to those of IMT. Some prepackaged CBT training modules may be purchased, but each will be different in its training effectiveness and its testing and data management requirements and capabilities (if any). Managing databases, data integrity, and reporting are difficult. In addition, keeping the functionality of the software updated is a major challenge, particularly ensuring continuity in the way content databases are structured and managed.

Web-Based Training

Increasing quantities of training materials are being offered on the Internet. These offerings are, in many cases, limited in scope and do not cover a broad set of topics. Users would need to monitor the availability of different topics, validate the author's credentials, and check to be sure the information is not outdated before the materials are used for training within an organization. Web-based training programs have varying levels of effectiveness, testing capabilities, and user management functions. It may be cumbersome to use Web-based training for organizationwide initiatives due to difficulties related to assigning group or individual lesson plans. Tracking or managing student test data may be even more difficult. All the numerous advantages of self-directed learning applications can accrue to the learner and the organization with Web-based training. However, the organization will need to have mechanisms in place to certify the curricula, assign lessons, track usage, and validate student test results.

Making the Final Decision

The ideal coding training program for CHW would need to cover all coding and compliance guidelines with comprehensive content delivery. To meet the coding training needs of CHW employees and managers, the program should allow for flexible lesson planning, tracking of student progress, and feedback on student performance with lesson plan adjustment capabilities.

Research showed that interactive computer-based coding training is probably just as effective as training provided through the classroom or lecture method. For example, on the coding portion of the AHIMA professional certification examinations, test candidates who learned to code using computer-based media had scores very similar to candidates who had learned coding through traditional classroom or group training (Scott and Bowman, 1998). Although computer-based coding training may lack the relational capabilities found in group training models, it can be an effective way to deliver didactic training. Ideally, computer-based training is supplemented with classroom, face-to-face training, or mentoring, to reinforce concepts or ideas.

Few health care organizations, including CHW, could bear the costs associated with the development of large-scale classroom training programs or internally developed self-learning methods. Of the electronic alternatives, the comprehensive computer-based curriculum approach using the Internet for delivery appeared to provide the most cost-efficient solution to the coding training challenges CHW's organizations faced. Ultimately, CHW senior executives, corporate compliance staff, and HIM directors chose to implement Web-based training. This training delivery format met more of the desirable attributes than any other learning method (see Table 10.2).

Since most of the coding training is of a technical nature and because the content must be updated regularly, Web-based training was viewed as the most cost-effective method for delivering consistent coding, medical terminology, and reimbursement education throughout the organization. Although some face-to-face educational sessions and mentoring of coders would be necessary for general compliance topics, Web-based training would allow the organization to target specific subjects and employee needs. This training delivery method would also fulfill the CHW goal of offering coding training to physician office personnel.

Coding practices are greatly influenced by ever-evolving federal and state reimbursement policies, published guidelines, and com-

Table 10.2. Desirable Attributes of a Systemwide Coding Training Program.

Desirable Attributes	Training Options			
	Manuals and Other Printed Training Media	Traveling Trainers	Computer-Based Training Modules	Web-Based Training
Flexibility	No	No	Yes	Yes
Around-the-clock availability	No	No	?	Yes
Administrator monitoring and oversight	No	Yes	Yes	Yes
Easy report production	No	No	?	Yes
Easy updates	No	?	Yes	Yes

Source: Adapted from D. K. Jones, *Compliance Accountability Training: Delivery Alternatives Compared.* WebInservice Enterprise Learning System: Concepts and Return on Investment. Atlanta, Ga.: MC Strategies, Inc., 2000.

plexities of private health plan reimbursement. Web-based training is an appropriate instruction delivery method when the training topics are subject to frequent or periodic change. Although Web-based training may be more expensive than printed materials or CD-ROM products, it is much easier to update the information in a Web-based program. For this reason, coding education using a Web-based training format seemed ideal.

The primary resistance to a Web-based training approach came from people concerned about the lack of face-to-face contact with an instructor. It was feared that learning might be stifled by the student's lack of direct give-and-take dialogue with a live coding teacher. One CHW hospital had developed an affiliation with a local community college coder training program and was concerned that this relationship might be jeopardized. These concerns did not undermine CHW's decision to seek out Web-based training solutions; however, everyone agreed that these issues should be monitored in the postimplementation evaluations.

There was also some fear that the Web-based training product would be the only mechanism that coders would have to learn about and enhance their coding knowledge. However, the CHW coding and HIM compliance program includes face-to-face in-facility workshops and three general seminars each year. The Web-based training product was intended to augment other learning techniques, not replace them.

Capacity Assessment

Before a final decision could be made about the instructional method that would be used to meet the goals of the coding education initiative, it was important to determine if CHW facilities had sufficient capacity to support Web-based training. Staff would need computers with Internet access. Bandwidth limitations might restrict instructional methodologies or slow performance.

A survey was conducted to determine whether the HIM departments in each CHW facility had access to the Internet. It was discovered that they did have access on at least one computer terminal. Therefore, access to Web-based training was possible for coders. Users of the Web-based training program could use the existing HIM department personal computers with Internet access or request that additional computers have access to the Internet. If the facility had an established computer-based training center, the coders could use this equipment for Web-based training. For the CHW clinic sites, it was discovered that the department managers had access to the Internet but staff access was limited. Before the coding training program could be rolled out to the clinics, decisions needed to be made regarding staff access to the Internet. This might involve adding additional computers or merely authorizing Web access for more of the existing computers.

Having a well-structured systemwide inventory of Internet accessible personal computers is very useful. Using the e-mail listings for employees, access and distribution lists were created for those currently using the Internet. Most of the people needing access to the Web for coding training or program administration already had Internet-accessible personal computers.

Another decision was to allow access to the Web-based training only through the CHW intranet. This decision was made in part because of legal advice but also because of the need to provide more structure and control of the training program. This decision will be reevaluated in late 2001, when the program has been in use for one year.

Internally Developed Versus Prepackaged Programs

Web-based learning systems are creating new educational opportunities in health care; however, these training programs can be very expensive to develop in-house. Companies must have dedicated systems and equipment; as well as staff knowledgeable in curriculum building, multimedia instructional design, and use of Web-authoring software tools. Dedicated staff would also be needed to update the training modules for topics that change periodically. If mediated feedback were a component of the training process, dedicated staff would be needed to provide students with this feedback. To justify these costs, a company must do a substantial amount of training (Lee and Owens, 2000).

CHW was not prepared to support an in-house Web training development initiative, and for this reason commercially developed Web-based coding training packages were investigated. The list of desirable attributes (Table 10.2) was used to evaluate vendor products. These requirements were unique to the needs of the CHW health system; the necessary features of Web-based training will vary according to the specific needs of any given facility or group of users. The criteria used by CHW are presented as an example and are not intended to establish an industry standard. It is unlikely that the entire list of features will be available in any one Web-based training product; however, the criteria serve as a starting point for discussions with vendors.

In the spring of 2000, the CHW director of coding and HIM compliance and several HIM department directors from CHW facilities evaluated Web-based coding training products available from these companies: American Health Information Management Association in Chicago, MC Strategies in Atlanta, and 3M Health Information Systems in Murray, Utah. CHW ultimately chose MC Strategies' WebInservice learning system for Web-based training. This learning system met the majority of our desired features. Training could be delivered throughout the health care system to hundreds of employees around the clock. Although the training is standardized, the system is flexible in that it allows for individualized lesson plans and focused study. The WebInservice system tracks employee learning progress and allows for competency testing. Most important, the WebInservice product includes high-quality coding lessons with content developed by qualified coding specialists. These learning modules are automatically updated to current national coding standards and guidelines. Learners have the ability to e-mail questions directly to the system administrator and other qualified coding resource consultants employed by MC Strategies. In addition, the company's long-standing history of quality computer-based coding education and its stable presence in the health care marketplace since 1986 were deciding factors for CHW.

Cost of Web-Based Training Products

It is important to understand that pricing may vary with vendor contract details, but overall savings can be achieved very quickly when comparing the cost of traditional education seminars or workshops with Web-based training products (see Table 10.3). For example, if one uses a $100 cost figure without other expenses, for attending six hours of coding education through seminar or workshop venues, this can easily translate to $2,666 per coder. To make this available to four thousand learners (staff), this equates to a $10 million price tag for systemwide coding education. Clearly, Web-based education is financially prudent for health care systems to employ.

Web-Based Training Phase-In Plan

A phase-in plan was devised to introduce the WebInservice learning system organizationwide. Evaluation and feedback would be provided at each step of the process. New categories of learners would be added to the system gradually. The proposed strategy was designed to be compatible with CHW's existing management structure, work processes, and technology infrastructure. Three key guidelines underscored the phase-in plan:

- Ensure that people are trained and oriented to use the Web-based learning system.

- Track to make sure that learners are using the system.

- Be sure that continual access to specific areas is covered by the focused lesson plans.

Table 10.3. Comparison of Costs: Face-to-Face Instruction Versus Web-Based Training for the CHW Coding Training Program.

Training Costs	Description	Approximate Cost of Face-to-Face Instruction (Six Hours, One Coder at One Facility)	Approximate Cost of Web-Based Training (Six Hours, One Coder at One Facility)
Training attendance costs	The expenditures associated with participant's time spent in training, travel, and per diem costs, and lost productivity or cost of replacing the individual while in training	6-hour seminar plus 2 hours travel time = 8 hours + 8 hours productivity time lost at $20 per hour = 16 × $20 = $320 *per trainee*	6 hours using the system + 0 travel time + 6 hours productivity time lost at $20 per hour = 12 × $20 = $240 *per trainee*
Instructor costs	The expenditures associated with instructor's time spent in training, travel, and per diem costs, and lost productivity or cost of replacing the individual while in training	6 hours training at $40 per hour = $240 per instructor. Travel costs = 2 hours at $40 per hour = $80 per instructor. Loss of productivity while training 3 hours at $40 per hour = $120 per instructor. Total: *$440 per instructor*	1 to 6 hours of training at $40 per hour = $40 *to* $240 *per instructor*
Instructional development personnel costs	The personnel expenditures during the design and development of the training materials	2 × 6 hours in class = 12 hours at $40 per hour = $480	1 to 6 hours of training at $40 per hour = $40 *to* $240
Additional instructional development costs	The nonpersonnel resources used during the design and development of the training materials	6 hours at $30 per hour = $180	1 to 6 hours of training at $40 per hour = $40 *to* $240
Facility, material, and equipment costs	Direct costs associated with delivery of the training	$10 per learner per 6-hour seminar	$0

The Web-based phase-in-training plan is illustrated in Exhibit 10.2. New groups of learners are brought into the project over an eight- to nine-month time period. Corporate leadership, headed by the corporate director of coding and HIM services, corporate compliance director, coding compliance specialists, ten CHW compliance officers, and the ten senior administrative representatives (CEOs, COOs, and CFOs), moved the implementation phases forward through the dissemination of information and benefits. Because approval for a CHW corporatewide initiative like this required high-level management approval, involvement of top management was central to moving the project forward.

Each HIM director guides the implementation and management within his or her hospital department and oversees staff compliance with the on-line program. The directors work with the appointed implementation staff at MC Strategies to arrange for the training needed to use the system. The directors have access to the facilities'

Exhibit 10.2. CHW's Web-Based Training Phase-In Plan.

Phase 1: Acute Care Hospital Coding Staff
- Inpatient coders
- Coding managers
- HIM coders for outpatient, ambulatory surgery, and emergency departments

Phase 2: Clinics and Home Health Agencies
- Coding staff
- Clinic managers
- Physicians

Phase 3: Case Managers and Utilization Staff
- Nurse case managers for inpatient and outpatient services

Phase 4: Patient Financial Services
- Billing service staff
- Business office staff
- Patient registration staff
- Admissions staff

Phase 5: Other ancillary or off-site areas where coding is conducted

WebInservice database in order to identify who is using the system and for how long, to obtain test results, and to ascertain other essential information.

Phase 1: Acute Care Hospital Coding Staff Implementation

In the fall of 2000, the Web-based coding training program was initiated at the CHW acute care hospitals. Implementation was rolled out in groups of six hospitals in a geographical cluster over a two- to three-week period. When one group ended the training period, the next six-hospital group started. Implementation began with conference call training to review the system functions and data management tools. Each site had a designated WebInservice administrator who was also part of the system implementation training. The entire Phase 1 implementation and training period for CHW acute care hospitals took twelve weeks (including time off for the year-end holidays).

Next Steps: Phases 2 Through 5

Phase 2 expanded the program to the CHW clinics (physician office staff) and home health agency personnel responsible for coding and data entry. Often staff in these clinical service delivery areas have coding reference books, but many have never received formal training in how to assign a code or apply coding principles. Informally trained coding staff tend to make coding errors in specialty areas. They may also be unaware of periodic code updates and changes and the impact of new governmental and private insurance requirements on coding and billing practices. The rollout plan for coding education in Phase 2 includes lesson plans for coding and billing staff in clinics and home health agencies. The clinic's designated lead supervisor assumed the role of WebInservice administrator. Phase 2 implementation in the clinics took two months to complete.

Case management and utilization staff will receive Web-based coding training in fundamental coding principles and clinical

documentation requirements in Phase 3. Armed with this knowledge, these staff will be better prepared to assist physicians in
maintaining accurate and complete documentation at the point
of patient care delivery. The case management directors at the
facility sites were asked to be the WebInservice administrators.
The time period for this phase was three to four months. The
implementation and training took several months as each of the
forty-eight acute care facilities had staff that needed training in
Phase 3.

During Phase 4, education and training will be expanded to people in financial services, business offices, patient registration units,
and admitting departments throughout CHW's network of health
care organizations. Medicare's implementation of an outpatient
prospective payment system with ambulatory patient classification
groupings makes it especially important that staff in these areas be
familiar with information capture and clinical documentation
requirements. Training in medical terminology and basic knowledge
of the coding systems will help these people do a better job in cap-
turing charges for services, supplies, and resource utilization so that
accurate code assignments can be made. The responsible staff for
this phase of the implementation will be the business office managers and the admitting supervisors. At the time of writing, this
phase had not yet been initiated. The estimated time frame for this
implementation is two months.

Phase 5 of the coding education and training program will
involve coding compliance training for ancillary service personnel,
such as those in radiology, lab, emergency rooms, and off-site entities such as wound care centers. Depending on their structure, these
ancillary areas from time to time require or provide coding services
to CHW. The ancillary area supervisors or managers will be responsible for implementation. The time frame for this is expected to be
two to three months, but at the time of writing this training had yet
to be initiated.

Evaluating Success

Evaluation of CHW's return on investment and management of the Web-based coding education will be evaluated at the user level and corporatewide. The following mechanisms that will be used to evaluate success and examples of performance measures:

- Hospital-specific feedback and reporting from the WebInservice learning system itself:

    Tracking of test-passing rates

    Tracking of problematic learning areas

- Expanded system utilization outside of HIM and success with using the system:

    Completion of specific assigned learning modules

    Tracking of test-passing rates

- Corporate tracking of CHW's implementation and utilization pattern:

    Completion of specific assigned learning modules by hospital group

    Completion of specific learning modules within given time frames

- Hospital-specific (internal) training development for specific staffing needs (for example, the "grow your own coder" program, which will assist with filling vacant coding positions):

    Number of successful coders completing the program

    Number of vacant coding positions filled by program-trained coders

- Corporate coding compliance identification of educational needs via compliance audits to feed into the Edu-Code module assignments on an ongoing basis

- Completion of systemwide implementation within one year of announcement to CHW staff

- Preparation of coding staff for national Certified Coding Specialist exam sponsored by AHIMA

- Tracking of communication to MC Strategies on coding content and lessons via Edu-Code's automated "light bulb" question-and-answer feature

- Calculation of system usage in hours and provision of feedback to corporate staff on financial value

- Determination of how the WebInservice learning system feeds into the individual coder's performance evaluation and how the information is used to identify areas needing improvement

The CHW corporate administrative team receives progress reports on a daily, weekly, monthly, and quarterly basis. These reports include data on the level of staff participation, staff receptiveness to the training program, actual individual progress on lesson completion, and overall adaptation of the training program within the work setting. A sample report comparing hospital usage is shown in Exhibit 10.3. The reports are produced through the WebInservice administrative report functions. The WebInservice administrator in each facility has the capability of generating reports directly off the learning system itself as it continuously tracks users and usage.

Initially, some people were concerned about the lack of face-to-face contact between students and instructors. To date, this has not proved to be a barrier to learning. People can interact with instructors via e-mail and also have the capability of discussing coding

Exhibit 10.3. Sample WebInservice Utilization Report.

Facility Name	Department	Lessons Assigned	Lessons Completed	Percentage Completed
Hospital A	9999	9	6	67
Hospital B	1111	9	9	100
Hospital C	5555	6	3	50

issues with other learners on the system or with their coding supervisor. Some concerns over content quality were identified, and MC Strategies addressed these directly and quickly. CHW staff also identified some features that needed changing, and the vendor responded to these recommendations within one month. The hospital with an affiliation with a community college coder training program had a positive outcome. Student on-the-job coding education supplemented with Web-based training provides a continuous feedback loop among coders, supervisors, and clinicians. This has resulted in improved coding quality.

Lessons Learned

Although implementation of the Web-based coding education program is in its early stages, CHW senior management has learned several lessons already. (1) The importance of selling the Internet-based technology as a learning method to directors and supervisors was greater than anticipated. (2) Concerns over the time needed to work on the system were also expressed, especially with current health care financial pressures (accounts receivable days and so on). (3) Close review of the curriculum content was identified as a need that required a collaborative effort between MC Strategies content specialists and the CHW corporate coding and HIM staff. (4) It is important for an organization to partner with internal information system staff; even though there is little work from their side, the sharing of information and overview of the project were found to be important and necessary. (5) Individual coding staff overall were very receptive, even eager, to use the system. (6) In addition, costs for staffing time to use the system must be clearly defined in advance to facilitate adjustments of departmental budgets and support systems.

CHW has had some early successes with the coding training program. One CHW facility has already trained three new coders using MC Strategies' WebInservice learning system. Every morning, the new employees participate in Web-based and paper-based coding instruction that includes simulated coding exercises. In the later part of the day, these new coders are given actual hospital records to code. After only three months into the learning process, the trainees exceeded the expectations of the HIM department director and facility management. The new coders are very enthusiastic about this accelerated on-the-job training process, and the results were well received by management. Another exciting benefit for CHW facilities located in rural areas is that new hires and existing coding staff now have access to ongoing and regularly updated coding education. CHW corporate leadership for the Web-based coder training program is sharing these positive benefits with the groups that will be involved in the later phases of the education rollout plan.

Meeting Your Needs Through Web-Based Training

We are all well aware that the government is recommending regular, ongoing compliance education for health care employees in high-risk departments. The employer needs to respond to this challenge with an organized and systematic implementation process. Having an educational initiative fall under the direction and leadership of corporate compliance can address specific needs of the coding areas and diminish potential risk. Upper management will need to demonstrate its commitment to this project and communicate its support.

The benefits of Web-based coder training and education should be trackable and reportable throughout the chosen system. Informational reporting is key to keeping track of the system, usage, and completion of any required lessons. The assignment of a site-specific system administrator provides a contact person for follow-up and clarification when needed.

Senior executives at CHW face staff training challenges for its coding staff. The CHW coding and HIM program brought the details of the issues to the table for discussion as a part of CHW's overall compliance program activities. Senior management was reminded that the Health Care Financing Administration strongly recommended ongoing education for high-risk staff like coders. Senior management was made aware that Web-based training could profoundly change the way clinical coding education was delivered across the CHW divisions and regions by the corporate director of coding and HIM compliance. This was achieved through live demonstrations, presentations, videoconferencing, and the dissemination of product literature. Web-based programs could also be used to assess the capabilities of current clinical coding staff and support career development and training of new coders.

Today's health care environment requires proactive programs to maintain and enhance the education and skill set of coding staff. Should you be providing easily accessible, consistent, and thorough training for your coding staff? This is a question that needs to be addressed by single health care facilities as well as multiple-setting health care delivery systems. Educational opportunities are now available in technology-based formats, and these formats offer training opportunities that never existed before. Health care organizations must learn how to transition from the more traditional training delivery models to Web-based training. Start this transition by establishing goals and objectives for moving into a Web-based training environment.

References

Lee, W. W., and Owens, D. L. *Multimedia-Based Instructional Design*. San Francisco: Jossey-Bass/Pfeiffer, 2000.

Office of the Inspector General, U.S. Department of Health and Human Services. *Compliance Program Guidance for Hospitals*. *Federal Register*, Vol. 63, No. 35, Feb. 23, 1998. [http://www.os.dhhs.gov/progorg/oig/oigreg/cpghosp.pdf].

Prophet, S. *Health Information Management Compliance: A Model Program for Healthcare Organizations*. Chicago: American Health Information Management Association, 2000.

Scott, K. S., and Bowman, E. D. *A Comparison of Traditional Methods Versus Computer-Assisted Instruction in Teaching Coding*. Chicago: American Health Information Management Association, 1998.

11

On-Target Education Program Meets Training Needs of Surgical Services

Alice T. Speers, Karen L. Zaglaniczny, Christine S. Zambricki

Challenges

- Lack of educational support
- Lack of formalized programs and standardized orientation
- Implementation of change
- Need to increase communication

Solutions

- Creation of education department staffed with multiskilled educators
- Development of competency-based orientation programs
- Development of internships, certification reviews, and continuing education programs
- Increased communication opportunities
- Creation of a learning environment

Results

- Improved compliance in the orientation process

- Staff participation in creative education programs

- Culture based on customer service excellence

- Better teamwork

- Appreciation of colleagues

William Beaumont Hospital in Royal Oak, Michigan, is a 997-bed major teaching and referral hospital that is the only Level I trauma center in Oakland County. It is one of the highest-volume providers, ranking first in the nation for inpatient admissions and first in Michigan for number of surgeries, births, and emergency visits. The hospital mission statement, "The patient is the center of all we do," guides the planning and provision of patient care services. The surgical services department at William Beaumont includes thirty-six operating rooms and ten procedure rooms with support for perianesthesia care of the patient.

The challenges facing our surgical services department began with the restructuring of the operating room in 1998 (see Figure 11.1). At that time, a new leadership team was recruited to improve our operating efficiency and expand services. This leadership team included directors for operating room services and the central processing department, perianesthesia services, information systems, and education and research.

The problems the surgical services faced in 1998 involved management, staffing, equipment, and education and training issues. People lacked confidence in the leader's ability to manage the high volume of cases seen in the department. Due to high attrition and poor staff retention, the surgical department had a chronic shortage of trained workers. The equipment problems included wrong, broken, or missing parts necessary for the surgical procedures.

Figure 11.1. Organizational Chart, Surgical Services, William Beaumont Hospital.

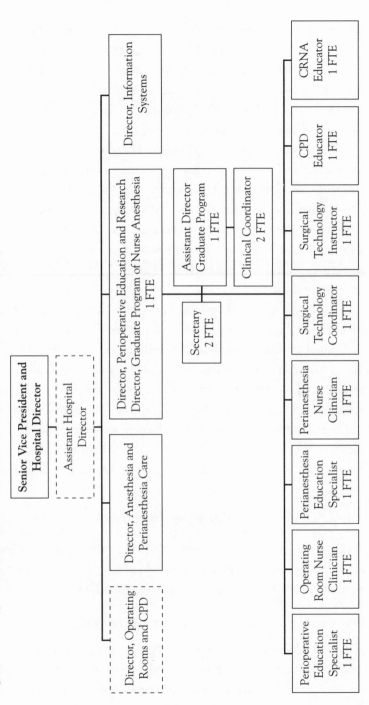

Education and training were minimal due to the lack of qualified educators and of instructional resources and inadequate time for staff orientation. In the initial education assessment of the department, the most compelling challenges identified were the decreased availability of qualified and skilled staff, lack of adequate orientation, insufficient resources, and the need for qualified educators.

The current orientation for registered nurses (RNs) and surgical technicians (STs) involved a two-week overview followed by assignments in the department. The turnover rate for staff was 40 percent. This high turnover appeared to be due to people's dissatisfaction with the working environment and lack of education and support. This high staff attrition rate had resulted in a downward spiral of workforce moral and a situation of staff shortages that seemed impossible to overcome.

Despite manpower shortages, the hospital's strategic plan called for continued growth in surgical services. In 1998, the department performed approximately forty-three thousand surgical procedures. To meet higher volume projections for the future, surgical services would need to expand hours and increase staffing. The hospital's ambitious expansion plans required creative educational initiatives in surgical services. The goal was to develop sound training programs that would ensure the surgical services at William Beaumont could provide top-quality patient care with knowledgeable and skilled staff.

Surgical Services Education Initiatives

To meet the surgical services expansion challenges at William Beaumont, many changes, new ideas, and exciting training programs were introduced. These initiatives are outlined here.

Perioperative Education and Research Department

A formal education department was created in surgical services to address the various staff training needs. This department is headed by a doctoral-prepared Certified Registered Nurse Anesthetist

(CRNA) director who is a member of the hospital nurse executive group and the operating room (OR) executive group. Staff in the department includes

Master's-prepared education specialists who are responsible for program development and evaluation

Baccalaureate-prepared nurse clinicians who are clinical experts in either the operating room or the perianesthesia care areas

Surgical technology instructors

A central processing educator

Master's-prepared educators for the CRNA staff members

A CRNA program director

The surgical services education department has been instrumental in developing, implementing, and evaluating the programs discussed in this chapter. The department has adopted the team concept to encourage continuous collaboration and sharing of resources. The education team participates in an annual planning retreat to identify and plan for future training needs in surgical services. There is a deliberate effort by all of the people in the education department to foster their own professional development by sharing their expertise with their peers and by participating in outside meetings and conferences. Each educator completes productivity logs (see Exhibit 11.1) to justify his or her workload and provide information for the director's use in discussions with hospital administration.

Operating Room Registered Nurse Internship Program

This twenty-four-week competency-based program prepares registered nurses with no previous OR experience to work as circulating nurses. The program consists of extensive didactic and clinical experiences that are based on AORN (Association of Perioperative

Exhibit 11.1. Perioperative Services Educator Workload and Productivity Log.

Name: _____   Week of: _____

Activity	Monday Calculate in minutes	Tuesday Calculate in minutes	Wednesday Calculate in minutes	Thursday Calculate in minutes	Friday Calculate in minutes	Weekly Total
RN/ST/CRNA/ORA/Medical Student Orientation Classes (teaching &/or coordinating)						
ORA Reorientation (teaching &/or coordinating)						
Clinical Orientation (scheduling, collaborating, evaluating)						
RN Internship/ST Program/Nurse Anesthesia Program Classes (developing, teaching &/or coordinating)						
Mandatory Education (scheduling, certifying/recertifying BLS, preparing for any mandatory session)						
Competency Validation (developing, checking level of competence)						
Inservice Education (coordinating &/or teaching)						
Continuing Education (developing program, obtaining approval, teaching &/or coordinating)						

Program Development (developing clinical or departmental program)							
Consultation (collaborating on clinical, educational, patient specific &/or operational issues)							
Strategic Planning (setting department goals, objectives, etc.)							
Support of Operations (time at routine standing meetings)							
Function Support (time spent assisting other educators at educational events)							
Conference Administration (time spent overseeing conference preparation)							
Patient Care (delivering direct patient care)							
Communication (group wise, phone messages, etc.)							
Travel (time spent traveling between department, OR, library, Nursing Education, and other work related areas)							

WEEKLY GRAND TOTAL =

Calculations: 8° work day = 7.5 hours × 60 minutes = 450 minutes   40° work week = 450 × 5 = 2,250 minutes

Source: Copyright © 2000, William Beaumont Hospital, Royal Oak, Michigan. Used with permission.

Registered Nurses) standards and recommended practices. The candidates participate in a series of interviews with the educators and managers who collaborate in the selection of the interns. The RN interns are hired into the program and receive all of the benefits of a full-time employee. They are promised a position upon completion and are required to commit to two years of service in the OR upon program completion. The results have been notable and positive.

Competency-Based Orientation

All newly hired RNs and STs with previous OR experience are provided with an individualized competency-based orientation of twelve to fifteen weeks. Operating room attendants and central processing technicians receive didactic and competency-based orientations in their respective areas.

Nursing staff in the perianesthesia care areas receive a competency-based orientation that focuses on the unique work in these areas. CRNA staff also participate in a competency-based orientation. It is important to note that all of the orientation plans incorporate the standards and recommended practices from each of the professional organizations.

Surgical Technology Programs

A "fast-track" surgical technology program was initially offered to meet an immediate need. The program consisted of classes and clinical experiences. The program was not accredited, however, and when graduation from a nationally accredited program became a prerequisite for ST certification, the hospital-based initiative was discontinued. An affiliation was forged with a local community college to offer an accredited associate degree program in surgical technology. Surgical technology educators from William Beaumont teach the college courses. Students gain clinical experience at William Beaumont and other hospitals affiliated with the college program.

Orientation Program Expansion

Prior to the development and implementation of the various OR internships and orientation programs, staff were afforded only a very brief introduction to this specialty area before they were sent out to fend for themselves and learn the best they could. When the internships were created, a commitment was made to the existing staff that they would also receive more education and clinical orientation into all of the OR specialties.

This one-year project involved eighty-five RNs and STs. Learning needs assessments were conducted and customized schedules were created to meet individuals' specific needs. Classes were provided in the basics, and a competency-based precepted clinical orientation was offered. Upon completion of the year, we were confident that our existing staff had solid baseline knowledge of the tenets of OR practices.

Surgical First Assistant Program

There is a great need for surgical first assistants, and very few educational programs are available. A surgical first assistant program has been developed at William Beaumont for OR certified registered nurses and certified surgical technologists. It is open to both internal and external applicants who meet the admission criteria (see Exhibit 11.2). The program contains both didactic and clinical components and is facilitated by the coordinator of the surgical technology programs. Content and clinical experts from William Beaumont teach the courses. The clinical component is the responsibility of the learner, as surgeon-monitored clinical experience in the role of the first assistant is required.

Certification Review Courses

At the time of the reorganization of surgical services in 1998, a commitment was made to encourage staff to become certified in their respective areas. To promote this initiative, review courses

Exhibit 11.2. Admission Criteria for the Surgical First Assistant Program.

- Transcripts from a nursing school, surgical technology school, or program verifying coursework in anatomy and physiology and microbiology with a passing grade of 2.0 or better. Registered nurses must show proof of a B.S.N. degree.

- A copy of current certification as a certified operating room nurse (CNOR) or certified surgical technologist (CST).

- Verification of employment verifying at least three years of full-time scrub experience or first assisting experience (or both) within the past five years.

- Proof of personal liability insurance covering activities as a first assistant.

- Proof of current cardiopulmonary resuscitation (CPR) or basic life support (BLS) certification.

- Results of a physical exam performed within the past three months and proof of current immunizations including those against hepatitis B and tuberculosis (or proof of exemption).

- References from two practicing surgeons who are familiar with the candidate's professional skills and can vouch for them and who also support the person's candidacy for the program.

- An essay (two hundred words or less, double-spaced) explaining why the candidate wants to be a surgical assistant.

have been developed for the OR staff (CNOR, certified OR nurse—see Exhibit 11.3—and CST, certified surgical technologist), central processing technicians, and the perianesthesia nursing staff (CPAN, certified postanesthesia nurse, and CAPA, certified ambulatory peri-anesthesia nurse). The programs are provided at no cost to employees and are offered at times and on days identified as convenient by the learners.

Basic Life Support Classes

The surgical services at William Beaumont have approximately seven hundred employees. It became apparent that because of its size, the department needed to be internally responsible for conducting basic life support classes and recertifications. The education department provides classes at the health care provider and "heartsaver

Exhibit 11.3. CNOR Review Program.

Class 1: Introductory Topics
AORN standards and practices
Nursing process
Patient education
Psychosocial aspects of OR nursing
Age-specific care
Test-taking strategies

Class 2: Physiological Monitoring Topics
Fluid and electrolyte balance
Acid-base balance
Anesthesia
Malignant hyperthermia
Preoperative care
Postoperative care

Class 3: Asepsis Topics
Aseptic technique
Sterilization
Sanitation
Skin preps
Surgical hand scrub
Gowning and gloving
Draping
Standard precautions

Class 4: Safety Topics
Positioning
Counts
Electrical safety
Chemical safety
Material safety data sheet
  (MSDS)
Fire safety
Laser safety
Latex allergy
Specimen handling
Pneumatic tourniquet

Class 5: Wound Closure and Instrument Topics
Skin integrity
Wound healing
Wound closure
Hemostasis
Infection
Care of instruments
Selection and evaluation of
  equipment

Class 6: Documentation Topics
Legal and regulatory requirements
Quality and performance
  improvement
Consents
Variance reports

Practice Test
200-item practice test

plus" levels for staff without current certification. Recertification sessions are also offered to staff whose certification is expiring. Both programs are provided on a quarterly basis and are taught by the perioperative educators.

Preceptor Program and Clinical Education

One of the basic tenets of the orientation programs is that a preceptor will guide the clinical experiences of new staff members. To maintain this philosophy, preceptors are needed in all of the clinical and support areas. Preceptors need a certain set of knowledge and skills; therefore, it was necessary to create and deliver a preceptor preparation program. This eight-hour class focuses on the principles of adult education, roles and responsibilities of the preceptor and the learner, creative strategies to deal with unique learners, documentation, and communication. The program is open to all staff members who meet preceptor selection criteria (see Exhibit 11.4) and are approved for a preceptor position by the manager. The basic preceptor preparation program is offered twice a year. It is approved for nursing continuing education credits. A clinical educator program for CRNA clinical instructors affiliated with the graduate and orientation program is offered annually.

Self-Directed Learning Materials and Modules

A variety of self-directed learning materials have been developed to meet specific learning needs of staff in surgical services. The learning materials are updated annually with the information needed to meet the mandatory education requirements of various regulatory and accreditation groups (see Exhibit 11.5). The self-directed learning materials, presented in a newsletter format, allow readers to review "the facts and only the facts" for various topics (see Exhibit 11.6). A multiple-choice test accompanies the materials. The completed tests are kept on file as proof of people's successful completion of the program.

Exhibit 11.4. Preceptor Selection Criteria.

Name: _____

Department: _____ Date of Completion: _____

Criteria	Met	Not Met
1. Employed in clinical area for at least 1 year with at least 6 months at Beaumont.		
2. Demonstrates competent practice in assigned work area.		
3. Demonstrates the ability to make deliberate and thoughtful decisions based on scientific and behavioral principles and thorough assessments.		
4. Exhibits team behaviors.		
5. Promotes positive, confidential interpersonal relationships through tactful, patient, direct, and sensitive interaction.		
6. Demonstrates a positive, professional attitude at all times.		
7. Demonstrates ability to provide both positive and negative feedback in a tactful manner.		
8. Demonstrates leadership skills in terms of setting priorities, making sound decisions, taking necessary risks, and being a role model.		
9. Demonstrates ability to introduce, interpret, and uphold protocols, policies, and standards.		
10. Demonstrates professional attributes in terms of performing work activities in a manner that maintains quality.		
11. Exhibits an interest in professional growth through participation in learning activities such as inservice programs, conferences, independent study, and continuing education.		
12. Demonstrates outstanding interpersonal and communication skills.		
13. Serves as a positive role model even during adverse, critical, or frustrating situations.		
14. Demonstrates willingness to share expertise with all learners regardless of classification.		
15. Creates and maintains an atmosphere that promotes learning and trust.		
16. States an interest in serving as a preceptor.		

Meets Criteria for Selection as a Preceptor: ❏ Yes   ❏ No

Manager: _____

Educator/Clinician:_____

Staff Member:_____

Source: Copyright © 2001, William Beaumont Hospital, Royal Oak, Michigan. Used with permission.

Exhibit 11.5. Excerpt from an Annual Education Update Table
of Contents.

Beaumont Standards

Customer Service Behaviors

Smoking

Oxygen Shut-Off

Wash Your Hands!

What Is the Quality Management Process?

Radiation Safety

Disaster Alert Codes

Informed Consent

Charting Guidelines

New "News" on Ergonomics

Security Tips for Personal Safety

Fire Safety in the Operating Room

Self-learning modules have been developed for the care of age-specific populations such as children and adolescents in the OR and perianesthesia care areas and the aging adult in the OR. The education department has prepared and distributed a self-directed module throughout the hospital on the topic of conscious (moderate) sedation. This module was developed in cooperation with the appropriate hospital nurse educators, CRNA educators, nurse managers, physicians, and performance improvement groups.

Continuing Education Offerings

In the state of Michigan, registered nurses must obtain continuing education credits in order to renew their license. Even though it is the responsibility of the individual nurse to accrue these credits, the surgical services education department provides educational programs that have been approved by the Michigan Nurses' Association for nursing contact hours. One day per week, surgical cases are started one hour later to allow time for staff education and business meetings. The educators plan an educational event twice a month

Exhibit 11.6. Excerpt from an Annual Update Learning Module on Personal Safety.

Security Tips for Personal Safety

The following tips will enhance your personal safety:

- Wear your WBH badge at all times and expect to see other employees wear their badge also.
- Make sure that your locker is securely locked before you leave the locker room—do not leave it open for a friend.
- Avoid carrying large sums of money. Keep car keys, credit cards, wallets, etc., separate from purses while going to and from your car.
- Plan your route of travel using well-lighted routes—walk with others if possible.
- Lock your vehicle and keep packages or other items out of sight

that relates directly to the care being provided in their respective areas. If the content is deemed to fit the criteria for continuing education credit, an application is made and contact hours are awarded. Over the span of a year, individual nurses are able to accrue continuing education credits pertinent to their daily work. In addition, educational programs are offered to CRNAs using outside speakers, case review, and research presentations. These allow CRNAs to obtain clinically relevant continuing education credits at the hospital.

William Beaumont is a Level I trauma center. To support this designation and provide surgical staff with perioperative trauma education, the department sponsors an annual perioperative trauma conference. The content varies from year to year and is based on a learning needs assessment that is completed by all staff in the various areas of the department, current needs, and special requests. The half-day conference is offered on a Saturday in the hospital auditorium to allow more staff to attend. It is offered at no cost to William Beaumont staff. The program is advertised in the community, and attendance and support from area hospitals has been overwhelming. The program has also been a small source of income for the education department in the form of vendor contributions and registration fees from outside participants.

Graduate Program of Nurse Anesthesia

In collaboration with Oakland University, William Beaumont developed the Graduate Program of Nurse Anesthesia in 1991. This twenty-eight-month full-time program results in a master of science degree in nursing and meets all of the national accreditation requirements. William Beaumont is the primary clinical site for students with didactic courses taught at the hospital and university. The hospital has benefited greatly from this program in terms of recruitment and retention. Approximately 47 percent of the students join the hospital staff following graduation. In anticipation of future expansion in surgical services at William Beaumont, class size has been increased from twelve to thirty students per year. An essential element of this, and any hospital-based education program, is the ability to flex the program in response to workforce needs.

Communication Initiatives

Communication in a large department in a very large health care institution can be challenging. Deliberate efforts have been made to improve communication within the surgical services department at William Beaumont. A bimonthly newsletter, fittingly named *The Cutting Edge,* provides information about the various programs, accomplishments, and special news in and around surgical services.

Staff meetings have been instrumental in providing a vehicle for sharing information. Each manager holds staff meetings twice monthly to address pertinent issues, concerns, changes, and suggestions for change. Every fifth Tuesday, a "town hall meeting" is held for all staff from all of the various subdepartments of surgical services. This meeting is led by the assistant hospital director responsible for surgical services and supported by the hospital director, the chief surgeons, and the directors of surgical services. It affords the surgical services staff members the opportunity to ask questions, seek clarification, share ideas for the future, and participate in the rollout of hospitalwide initiatives.

Managers attend a weekly surgical services management meeting to keep abreast of changes, news, and plans for the future. One of these meetings is dedicated to discussing specific concerns between the educators and managers. It has helped form a strong alliance between these two complementary groups.

Communication is a two-way street. Multiple processes have been initiated to ensure that staff can easily communicate with surgical services administration. Beyond our open-door policy for management, suggestion boxes have been installed throughout the surgical areas. The suggestions are reviewed and discussed at the management meeting, and the responses are reported in *The Cutting Edge*. An anonymous hotline for telephone reporting of concerns or potential safety issues has also been established.

The educational needs in the surgical services department have been great, and the response has been rigorous. The task will continue as surgical services are expanded with the construction of sixteen additional operating rooms and ten procedure rooms over the next three years. In addition, increased technological complexity and the never-ending need for qualified staff will require strong educational support.

Value of Internal Educational Efforts

The hallmark of the exceptional educational initiatives in the surgical services department at William Beaumont is increased satisfaction among our patients, surgeons, staff, management, and administration. Patient and surgeon satisfaction surveys have consistently demonstrated ratings of excellence. Staff are highly complimentary of the educational opportunities and the sound, competency-based orientation process. Staff member orientation is individualized and based on the experience level of the staff. This has been a valuable recruitment strategy. Managers and administrators are impressed with the accomplishments that are evident in the daily functioning of the department. Educational offerings and programs are provided to all employees at no cost. The surgical services department has been able to expand to meet the demands of an ever-increasing patient population.

Our RN internship model has been adopted by other hospital departments (including critical care, medical nursing, the cardiac catheterization laboratory, and the family birth center) to use in training staff members. The development and implementation of a surgical technology program offers a career ladder for other employees in the hospital. The exemplary collaborative efforts for interdisciplinary education have contributed to the personal and professional growth of the surgical services education team.

Although the surgical services department has experienced many positive outcomes from the educational initiatives, there have been some confrontations. One of the most significant challenges was the need to implement change. Staff members were skeptical about the ambitious educational initiatives and voiced concerns as to how anything could be different when staffing and morale were so low. Managers were frustrated when they could not use orientees to fill staff vacancies. Through daily reassurances, involvement of staff, and evidence of the commitment to change, improvements were noted and celebrated.

A perceived disadvantage to the institution was the extensive financial costs involved in recruitment, staff education, program development, implementation, and evaluation. Hospital administration invested a tremendous amount of financial and resource support. The results have been tremendous, as evidenced in the successful expansion of surgical services, education, retention of staff, and most important, quality of patient care. Education is a priority throughout the corporation and continues to receive support.

Although the emphasis for creating a learning environment has contributed positively to employee satisfaction, the system is not a panacea. For example, on the last employee survey, staff members reported that improvements are needed in the area of employee recognition.

Lessons Learned

Many lessons were learned during the development and implementation of educational initiatives in the surgical services department. These lessons dealt with issues surrounding the development of a culture based on customer service excellence for patients, surgeons, staff, and leaders. Paramount to this excellence is the need for teamwork, collaboration, and appreciation of all involved. Managers, staff, and educators must be involved in developing and implementing programs. Orientation of all staff must be competency-based, individualized, and founded on professional standards. Recognition of the fact that not all staff want to be educated and trained requires "win them over" efforts. This was effectively accomplished through listening, counseling, and persistence. The benefits of interdisciplinary support and sharing have promoted tremendous learning opportunities.

All of the surgical services' educators demonstrate team spirit and a willingness to help colleagues throughout the department. The educators have been a valuable resource in networking with other departments and hospitals. In return, the surgical services department has benefited by learning and implementing new ideas, practices, and strategies.

The efforts of the education and management teams have been tireless and will continue. The commitment to service expansion and top-quality patient care will require regular evaluation and revision of our education programs to meet the needs of staff members. Change is ongoing, and we will continue to face the challenge.

12

· ·

Education Collaborative Augments Staff Training in Northern California Hospitals

Rebecca Petersen

Challenges
· ·

- Staff shortages in many health care occupations have created workforce training and education challenges for individual hospitals.

- Hospitals, by themselves, cannot meet all the educational needs of new hires and existing staff.

Solutions
· ·

- Form an educational collaborative among hospitals in Northern California to provide training that individual hospitals do not have the faculty or time to teach.

- Create opportunities for skill development and workforce training that are available to a wide range of health care professionals.

Results
· ·

- Increased ability for hospitals to meet staff training needs without substantial expenditures

- Flexible training opportunities for health care professionals in the Northern California region

• Regional collaboration among health care providers to
solve recruitment and staff development challenges

Health care organizations have weathered staffing shortages in the
past; however, many hospital executives were unprepared for the extent of the current situation. Numerous factors have contributed to
what is being called in California a "public health crisis." Registered
nurses and allied health professionals, many of whom are now in
their late forties and early fifties, are retiring or preparing to do so.
Enrollment in nursing and allied health educational programs is
down. Difficult-to-replace school faculty are retiring. Importing
nurses and staff from other states or countries is not the option it
once was because shortages are now so widespread. Some people in
California blame the technology industry for the staff shortages
in health care. Young people are lured to jobs with promises of high
pay, stock options, and a work environment that does not contain
bloodborne pathogens, bedpans, understaffing, or night shifts.

New graduates are entering hospital environments where
resources are scarce, patients are very sick, and mentors and clinical educators are almost nonexistent. There simply isn't enough
time to thoroughly train nurses and other allied professionals before
they are thrown into the fray. Often newly graduated nurses are
hired directly into specialty units such as critical care or the emergency department. The competition to hire these new graduates is
fierce, and there are often lavish incentive packages to entice them.
It is all too common for hospitals to invest in orientation and training only to have staff lured away to "better" positions elsewhere.

Support technical staff members are being trained to do other
jobs. For instance, emergency medical technicians are being cross-
trained to work as monitor technicians in telemetry units or as EKG
technicians. Nursing assistants are being trained to do other jobs
also, including central service instrument processing, EKGs, and
phlebotomies.

Unfortunately, many health care organizations are downsizing education services at a time when there is a greater need than ever for cross-training and ongoing staff education. A minimum number of education staff are responsible for providing new employee orientation and for conducting the in-service training required by regulatory agencies and accreditation groups. The position of clinical nurse specialist has been all but eliminated in many facilities, despite the fact that people in that position perform an important education role, providing orientation for new nurses as well as specialty training for existing staff. Managers are often responsible for multiple units and therefore do not have the opportunity to guide and groom new employees and new graduates; day-to-day management and staffing issues consume much of their time. Strategic educational issues are hard to solve when managers are overwhelmed by the task of finding staff to work the next shift.

Easing Training Challenges Through Collaboration

The education and training issues facing health care organizations today cannot be easily solved at the institutional level. Collaborative efforts among providers and other institutions are needed. In Northern California, this collaborative effort has already begun under the umbrella of the Hospital Consortium Education Network (HCEN), an arm of a not-for-profit corporation, the Hospital Consortium of San Mateo County (HCSMC). Founded in 1983, the corporation began as a venture of five independent hospitals as a vehicle for conducting business that was mutually beneficial and noncompetitive. Those hospitals were Mills Hospital in San Mateo, Peninsula Hospital in Burlingame, Sequoia Hospital in Redwood City, Seton Medical Center in Daly City, and San Mateo County General Hospital in San Mateo. The consortium supported several activities, including a centrally located education center for use by employees at the five hospitals.

In 1995, the HCEN was formed to strengthen the educational branch of the HCSMC. To accomplish the goal of offering educational services to as many facilities in the San Francisco Bay Area as possible, a new training facility was constructed in Pleasanton and nonprofit hospitals were offered HCEN membership. Initially, local hospitals were targeted for membership; however, as the benefits of the education collaboration became more publicized, hospitals from throughout Northern California began to take part. Today more than fifty hospitals are members. The HCEN has also developed affiliations with other education-oriented groups such as the Northern California Training Institute, the training arm of the AMR Ambulance Company.

The HCEN has grown rapidly. The organization now has fifty-three sponsoring members, which include hospitals, Samuel Merritt College, and the fire departments of Alameda County. Training class participation has increased from 3,926 in fiscal year 1994–95 to 9,875 in fiscal year 1999–2000. Revenue has gone from $480,000 in 1994–95 to $1,353,000 in 1999–2000. Average class size today is fourteen (classes are often held even if there are only five or six people in attendance).

The Early Days

Prior to the formation of the HCEN, the HCSMC provided education programs in the consortium offices in Burlingame, just south of San Francisco International Airport. Nurse educators from the five founding hospitals came to these facilities to teach classes. The hospitals paid these educators' salaries. Training session participants were charged tuition to cover HCSMC overhead costs. To expand the education offerings, experts from specific fields were recruited to teach. More people began to sign up for training from organizations outside the founding hospitals. A tiered fee schedule was developed in which participants from member hospitals paid less than those from outside the HCSMC. The demand for education from both member and nonmember hospitals increased significantly, and the HCSMC soon realized that it had reached the saturation point for the number of people willing to drive to the central training facilities. In 1995, the decision was made to grow the education initiative by increasing the scope of services and widening the geographical range. A new full-time director of education services was hired, and the HCEN was formed as a distinct entity. The structure of the HCEN and its relationship to the HCSMC are illustrated in Figure 12.1.

Figure 12.1. Structure of the Hospital Consortium of San Mateo County (HCSMC) and the Hospital Consortium Education Network (HCEN).

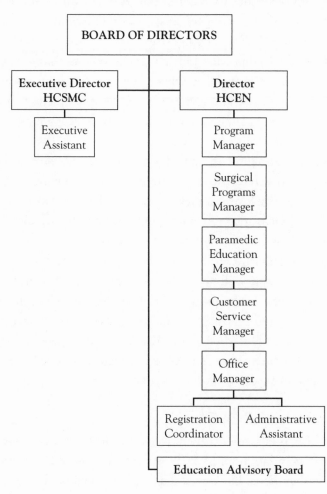

The ability to offer sponsoring memberships was a key component in the HCEN strategic plan. Without changing the ownership structure of the corporation, the formation of a separate entity under the umbrella of the consortium allowed hospitals from throughout the Bay Area the opportunity to join the education network.

The goal of the HCEN is to assist member hospitals in their efforts to deliver high-quality staff education. Although formal affiliation agreements are in effect, the HCEN does not interfere with the decision-making authority of the individual facilities. Initially, the concept of an education consortium was met with some fear by the education staff at prospective sponsoring hospitals. Some people viewed the HCEN as competition or as a threat to their job. Over time, the facility education staff have come to realize that the HCEN philosophy is one of assistance, not takeover. Joint planning, shared goal setting, and ongoing assessment of results help ensure the effectiveness of HCEN support. If facilities already have internal or external training systems in place, the HCEN does not attempt to disturb those systems. There is a conscious effort to build a positive, win-win relationship with each sponsoring member and to ensure that employees at member facilities have access to needed education services and problem-solving consultations. Sponsors can continue to use their own internal resources for education, with the HCEN providing the services that are not cost-effective for one organization to offer alone. This has eliminated many of the job security concerns for hospital education employees. The education staff at sponsoring organizations now have even more educational resources available to them. The HCEN can design classes specifically for an organization or can bring in already developed programs to the sponsoring sites.

Education Advisory Board

The HCEN is customer-driven. Representatives from sponsoring member organizations provide direction on the specific educational offerings they would like to see. An education advisory board, made up of representatives from member facilities, meets quarterly to guide the HCEN's educational priorities. At these board meetings, people discuss training needs that are not being met by individual hospitals but that may be met by the HCEN. The advisory board provides direction for the HCEN, monitors quality and utilization of training programs, proposes new programs, and works together in a noncompetitive environment to solve problems common to all members, such as recruitment and retention issues. Recruitment challenges were what prompted the development of the HCEN Registered Nurse Refresher Program. An executive committee of the advisory board drafted an outline of the curriculum for this twelve-day program. The draft was circulated to the entire board, which made suggestions that were incorporated into the final design (see Exhibit 12.1). This consensus process is used often as the HCEN refines and redesigns programs to keep the education offerings current.

Composition of the membership for the education advisory board has been a challenge. Each hospital chooses one or more

Exhibit 12.1. RN Refresher Course Curriculum.

Day 1:	Overview of the Changes in Health Care
Day 2:	Scope of Practice
Day 3:	Physical Assessment
Days 4 and 5:	Drug Review
Day 6:	IV Refresher
Day 7:	Nutrition and Wound Care
Day 8:	Pain Management: The Fifth Vital Sign
Day 9:	Infectious Diseases
Day 10:	Lab and Diagnostics
Day 11:	Skills Review (hands-on practice with IV sticks, tubes and drains, glucose monitor, PCA pump, infusion pump, pumps for external feeding, Code Blue, oxygen delivery devices, suctioning, and Dynamap)
Day 12:	Putting It All Together

representatives. Initially, the facility's senior education decision makers—the chief nurse executive and human resource manager—were encouraged to be on the board. However, over time, board membership has evolved to a very diverse group. Today, membership includes chief nurse executives, education directors, clinical nurse specialists, and education coordinators. Kaiser Northern California is a sponsor and represents fifteen hospitals. Different people from both the Northern and Southern California divisions attend board meetings. Their perspective serves to enrich and enhance meetings. Occasionally, it would be helpful if more senior staff from member hospitals attended the board meetings, especially when financial decisions are being made regarding programming priorities. For the most part, however, a diverse membership helps everyone see the issues from different vantage points, which is a valuable learning experience.

Benefits of Sponsoring Membership

By offering hospitals sponsoring membership, the HCEN was able to greatly expand the geographical area in which classes are offered without the need to rent classroom space. Benefits for the hospitals are enormous and have increased over time. Sponsors pay no membership fees. Revenues for the HCEN come exclusively from class tuition. Sponsoring members must agree to three provisions:

- To host a minimum of three classes per year on-site at their facility. Organizations that cannot meet this requirement must pay an annual fee of $1,500. To date, no members have elected to do this.

- To provide classroom space sufficient to accommodate at least twenty students and audiovisual equipment.

- To schedule classes (that are open to outside participants) far enough in advance for inclusion in the HCEN class catalogue, published three times per year.

In return for sponsoring membership, the organization receives the following services and benefits from the HCEN:

- Discounted tuition for employees for all classes taken at any HCEN location. There are further discounts when classes are held on-site at the member's facility and even further discounts if the facility is paying the tuitions for its participants (see the fee schedule in Exhibit 12.2).

- Marketing of classes to employees through course catalogues and flyers. The HCEN catalogue is extensive and offers a vast array of programs. In addition, brochures are produced for longer training programs. The brochures outline class prerequisites and application procedures as well as curriculum and expectations for completion of the programs. The course catalogue and brochures are also on the Internet at the HCEN web site (www.hospitalconsort.org). Participants can register for classes on-line. A strategic goal of the HCEN is eventually to offer some on-line classes.

Exhibit 12.2. Education Fee Schedule for a Regular One-Day Class.

Member: $110 ($100 if registration is received two weeks in advance of the class)

Nonmember: $90 ($80 if registration is received two weeks in advance of the class)

- If a class is held at a sponsoring site, the employees of that organization pay $65. Other participants pay the regular rates.
- If a class is being paid for by the sponsoring organization and the class is held on-site, a sliding-scale fee schedule applies. Rates may vary, depending on course content and the number of instructors needed, but generally the fees are as follows:

1–20 participants: $1,000 per day
21–30 participants: $1,300 per day
31–40 participants: $1,500 per day

- Continuing education records of participants and information about employees who have attended a particular program. For instance, if surveyors from an external accreditation group want to know how many people have taken a class in pediatric assessment, the HCEN can provide a list of employee participants and the date the program was completed.

- Recognition as a sponsoring organization on all HCEN promotional materials, catalogues, and stationery. This creates a great sense of ownership and encourages participation.

- The opportunity to participate in an institutional staff educational assessment that includes a detailed summary and recommendations. The HCEN will design a survey in conjunction with the organization. The organization distributes the survey to employees. Completed surveys are returned to the HCEN, which tabulates and analyzes the results. Based on the survey findings, the HCEN provides the organization with recommendations for classes that could be scheduled at the facility.

- Opportunities for the sponsor's employees to teach classes. Faculty from sponsoring organizations are encouraged to teach for the HCEN. They get to keep their teaching skills sharp, meet clinical ladder requirements, apply their expertise in a different setting, and contribute to the overall success of the educational consortium.

- Membership on the HCEN educational advisory board to assist in setting education priorities for program offerings.

HCEN Educational Offerings

Each quarterly HCEN catalogue includes approximately 350 days of education programming for health care professionals. These classes are held at the HCEN training facilities and in the classrooms of sponsoring members. Exhibit 12.3 shows a sample listing of the topics covered in one quarter. In addition to addressing the general training needs of nursing staff, the HCEN offers many courses of interest to nurses and other people working in areas such as critical care, emergency departments, neonatal intensive care, labor and delivery, management and leadership, case management, and quality management.

To facilitate entry or reentry for health care professionals and provide opportunities for people to advance in their profession, the HCEN sponsors longer training programs for surgical technologists, perioperative nursing, central service technicians, anesthesia technicians, and phlebotomists. The HCEN also has an RN refresher course and new RN graduate orientation. To increase the number of available workers, the National Council Licensure Examination (NCLEX) review course is offered to help nurses, especially those who were trained abroad, to pass the Registered Nurse exam. This is especially important in a state where there are a high number of foreign-trained nurses and where the licensure exam pass rate for these individuals is quite low.

The HCEN addresses the needs of nursing assistants by offering a menu of courses specifically designed to meet their continuing education requirements at a reduced price. A special brochure is printed and mailed to the nursing assistants in the HCEN database and to the education departments of hospitals throughout Northern California. Certified nursing assistants are encouraged to take classes to improve and enhance their careers.

A wide variety of allied health professions gain educational assistance from the HCEN. For radiology technicians, the HCEN has a

Exhibit 12.3. Sample Table of Contents of an HCEN Course Catalogue.

ACLS Preparation
ACLS Provider and Instructor
Antepartum Nursing
Bedside Emergencies
Blood Withdrawal Certification
Cancers of Men and Women
Cardiac Drugs and Drips
Charge Nurse Skills
Chemotherapy
Communication Skills
Conscious Sedation
Critical Care Certification
Critical Thinking
Cultural Health Perspectives
Dealing with Difficult People
Defusing Assaultive Behavior
Dementia
Diabetes Update
Diet, Food, and Mood
Director of Staff Development
EKG: Basic, Advanced, 12-Lead
Emergency Medical Technician
  Refresher
Emergency Nurse Pediatric Course
End of Life
Ethical Issues
Fetal Heart Monitoring
Fluids and Electrolytes
Forensic Nursing
Geriatric Assessment
Hemodynamic Monitoring
Hepatitis A–G
HIV/AIDS
Infectious Diseases
Informed Consent
Intra-Aortic Balloon Pump
Intrapartum Complications
IV Administration Update

IV and Contrast Medium Skills
  for X-Ray
IV Therapy Certification
Joint Replacement
Labor and Delivery Certification
Laboratory Tests
Latex
Leadership Certification
Leadership Symposium:
  Ethics in the Workplace
Legal Issues in Documentation
Legal Issues in Nursing
Medical Nutritional Therapy
Medical Terminology
Menopause
Monitor Technician Training
National Council Licensure Exam
  Review
Neonatal Resuscitation
Neurological Assessment
Nursing Research
Nutrition
Pain Management
Physical Assessment
Psychiatric Assessment
Psychopharmacology
Quality Management
Renal Failure
Respiratory Assessment
Respiratory Disease Management
RN Refresher Certification
Robots in the Operating Room
Spanish for Health Care
Trauma
Trauma Nurse Core Curriculum
Tuberculosis
Vascular Nursing
Ventilator Workshop
Wound Care

Abbreviations: ACLS, Advanced Cardiac Life Support; EKG, Electrocardiogram;
IV, Intravenous.

training program in intravenous (IV) and contrast media skills to train people in IV line insertion technique and enhance their knowledge of the allergenic properties of contrast media. Students perform two intravenous sticks in class and perform eight more under physician supervision before certification is granted. The HCEN offers a number of classes for respiratory care practitioners, including respiratory assessment, respiratory disease management, mechanical ventilation, and specialty care topics such as respiratory therapy for patients in neonatal intensive care. The needs of marriage, family, and child counselors and of licensed clinical social workers are met through HIV/AIDS programs and age-specific assessment and gender-specific programs. These programs are also helpful for other disciplines, as are HCEN courses in stress management, defusing assaultive behavior, dealing with difficult people, infectious diseases, diabetes updates, nutrition, and wound care. At the request of San Mateo County and the San Mateo Fire Departments, the HCEN has developed paramedic training courses.

The HCEN offers Spanish classes for health care providers. These classes have been very well received in California, a state where Spanish is one of the primary languages spoken. The HCEN also offers a special program on cultural health perspectives in the Latino community to assist sponsoring members in educating all members of their health care team in cultural competencies.

The six-day management leadership program is designed for everyone on the management team. This program is often used by hospitals for team building and collective problem solving. Areas of major focus for the Joint Commission on Accreditation of Healthcare Organizations are covered in the HCEN programs on patient restraint, documentation, pain management and patients' rights, advance directives, and informed consent.

The HCEN's educational offerings continue to be refined and redesigned based on input from the educational advisory board and the needs of health care professionals and providers in Northern California.

HCEN Faculty

The faculty for HCEN programs come from several sources, including universities, specialty practices, and nursing schools. Most are independent contractors who teach at the HCEN part time. A few hospital-based nurses complete their clinical ladder requirements for staff nurse III designation by teaching courses for the HCEN. It can sometimes be difficult to find sufficient numbers of preceptors for programs that require a clinical component. The HCEN tries hard to recognize people who serve as preceptors. Some facilities allow us to pay preceptors a modest honorarium; others request that the HCEN donate to the hospital's education fund. In some instances, delivery of a basket of gourmet coffee and bagels makes the preceptors feel appreciated.

Lessons Learned and Challenges Ahead

Since its inception in 1995, the HCEN has learned many important lessons about creating a successful educational collaboration among health care organizations. It has been essential to stay focused on common educational concerns, which can sometimes be difficult to do when competitors collaborate. The HCEN works closely with member hospitals and communicates frequently. Through the advisory board, members select and design the HCEN's courses according to their needs and standards. Such involvement creates the sense of ownership and commitment needed to keep the HCEN functioning. Sponsoring members realize that they cannot, by themselves, meet all the educational needs of staff. The HCEN is viewed as an important resource for education programs that sponsors do not have the time or the faculty to teach.

Several issues continue to be challenging. Student fees can sometimes be barriers. Class prices are negotiable, as many of our sponsors have learned. There is never a time when something can't be worked out to everyone's satisfaction. For example, a hospital might bargain for slots in an Advanced Cardiac Life Support class in exchange for providing clinical experiences for an HCEN student enrolled in a training program such as perioperative nurse training or paramedic training.

Perioperative training is currently the area of greatest difficulty for the HCEN. In response to the enormous shortage of operating room nurses, in 1998 a pilot training program aimed at registered nurses with two years' acute care experience was developed. Members of the education advisory board helped guide the planning for this six-month, three-day-a-week program. The first class enrolled and graduated ten nurses. The program was evaluated and revised, based on lessons learned from the pilot. Subsequent classes have remained small and have not been financially successful (barely breaking even or losing money). Sponsoring members agree this is a high-caliber training program that should be continued. The tuition is only $4,500; however, nurses enrolled in the program also expect to be paid their regular salary during the training. This adds another $30,000 to $40,000 to the hospital's costs, thus making it prohibitive for most budgets.

It is also hard to recruit experienced nurses for the training. Many nurses are unfamiliar with the career opportunities in perioperative services, especially now that nursing schools do not routinely offer an operating room rotation. When a perioperative nurse retires, the hospital is at least one year away from having a fully trained replacement (six months in the HCEN program and six months of on-the-job training). Some of our sponsoring members are already canceling elective surgery cases because of staff shortages. Operating room nurse staffing is a critical issue that needs the attention of senior executives. It can't be solved at the managerial level in most organizations.

For the HCEN, recruiting students and preceptors for the perioperative training program remains a challenge. A total of sixty-eight perioperative nurses have been trained so far in six classes. Because the need for perioperative nurses is so great in Northern

California, the HCEN plans to continue the training and to subsidize those courses from other more lucrative programs if necessary.

Another HCEN program in the surgery area is surgical technician training. In 1995, the HCEN was conducting the only accredited nonmilitary surgical technician-training program in Northern California. This highly successful program was taught full time for ten months and included six months of clinical operating room rotations in two participating hospitals. After ten years, the program maintained a perfect record in scores on the national certification exam: 100 percent of graduates passed the exam. This program had another advantage in that the HCEN was able to offer it in collaboration with a local community college. Students were registered at the college and received all the benefits, including counseling and library services as well as credit toward an associate degree. Unfortunately, the HCEN was unable to enroll a sufficient number of students in 2000 to hold the program. Applications for the program have decreased over the past few years, and in 2000 the number of applicants was minimal. This was surprising. Although many new surgical technician training programs had sprung up in Northern California, they are more expensive and are not accredited. In trying to determine why the HCEN program no longer attracted applicants, we reached the following conclusions:

- Students experienced great difficulty trying to finance a ten-month full-time program that resulted in a fairly low-paying job (about $13 per hour).

- Some of the other training programs had marketing budgets that allowed greater visibility than the HCEN program.

- After ten years, the HCEN had placed over one hundred surgical technicians in the immediate area, and job openings were fewer.

- The HCEN had begun to place more emphasis on training nurses for the perioperative role.

There were also issues with the community college with regard to fees. It became increasingly difficult for the college to justify the tuition students paid to the HCEN in addition to the community college enrollment fees, even though the net result was a training course far less expensive than any other. Because the HCEN failed to offer the surgical technician training program in 2000, the community college has taken over the program and will seek independent accreditation status. Although this is a loss for the HCEN, it is a lesson we can learn from as other programs are instituted.

Collaboration Benefits

While the HCEN continues to struggle with some educational issues, it continues to provide a unique solution to the training challenges confronting hospitals in Northern California. It is a collaborative model that can be adapted to other locations and has enormous potential for organizations seeking cost-effective training options. There are few limits to the education programs that the HCEN can offer. With increased use of the Internet, new populations of students can be reached. The implications for rural health applications alone are tremendous.

Hospital collaboration is the key to success in staff education, and education is a way to reduce the workforce shortages in many health care occupations. The big question among many baby boomers is, "Who will be at the bedside to care for me in the not too distant future?" Through careful use of resources and collaboration in education, the HCEN and other collaborative systems based on the same model will provide part of the answer.

During the next ten years, collaborative models for education services can reach greater numbers of people and provide economies of scales for health care systems as well as independent hospitals. By allowing an organization such as the HCEN to design facility-specific programs in this time of rapidly changing needs gives every participant an advantage.

Using new technologies, the HCEN will be able to reach more people and combine teaching techniques in ways never before thought of while maintaining the foundation of classroom instruction. Hands-on skills training will be more important than ever as we find new ways to manage patient care cost-effectively. By continuing to respond to members' needs, the HCEN will continue to grow and become even more valuable to the health care communities it serves. Our goal is to be the provider of choice for health care education in Northern California. The HCEN is also seeking opportunities to replicate the model in Southern California and in other states. For more information, see the HCEN's Web site at www.hospitalconsort.org.

Glossary

· ·

The Language of Learning

abilities   Attitudes, characteristics, or attributes that a person needs to possess to perform a job task.

attendance costs   The expenditures associated with a participant's time spent in training, travel to the training site, and lost productivity or cost of replacing the individual while in training.

competence   Demonstrable behaviors and characteristics that identify discrete levels of performance based on established criteria.

competency   A cluster of related knowledge, skills, and other attributes that affect a major part of one's job that correlates with performance on the job, can be measured against well-accepted standards, and can be improved via training and development.

effectiveness   The level of achievement of program goals and the results intended (for example, "percentage of reduction in medication administration errors").

instructor costs   The expenditures associated with an instructor's time spent in training, travel to the training site, and lost productivity or cost of replacing the individual while in training.

Kirkpatrick's evaluation model   A four-level model of training evaluation that allows the measurement of different training outcomes, including participant reactions, learning, on-the-job behaviors, and organizational results.

knowledge   The facts, concepts, and principles needed to perform a job task.

learning organization   An organization that expects change and prepares its employees to achieve success in a dynamic work environment.

learning style   How learners respond to a variety of learning experiences. The three key learning styles are visual, auditory, and tactile.

monitoring   Consistently measuring performance and providing ongoing feedback to employees and work groups on their progress toward reaching training objectives.

motivation   Processes or conditions that can energize and direct a person's behaviors in ways intended to gain rewards or satisfy needs.

needs assessment   A determination of priority training needs either now or in the future.

outcomes   The results of a training activity compared to its intended purpose.

performance   Observable actions or behaviors reflecting the knowledge or skill acquired from training to meet a task demand.

performance goal   A target level of performance expressed as a tangible, measurable objective, against which actual achievements can be compared, indicating a goal expressed as a quantitative standard, value, or role.

planning   Setting performance expectations and goals for groups and individuals to channel their efforts toward achieving training objectives.

return on investment A comparison of the costs of training to the savings or other financial benefits derived as a result of training.

rewarding Recognizing employees, individually and as members of groups, for their performance and acknowledging their contributions to the organization's mission.

self-directed learning A process by which an individual takes responsibility for his or her own training in partnership with the employing organization. The individual contributes a real and personal commitment to learning, acceptance of responsibility, and self-discipline. The organization contributes such real factors as the opportunity (time and attitude) for learning and competence development, feedback, and equipment and resources (publications, multimedia, assignments, details, and so on).

skill An organized and coordinated act or task designed to achieve a specific goal. Can also be a qualitative expression of performance, for example, how well an individual accomplishes the act or task.

staff development Increasing employees' capacity to perform through training, giving assignments that introduce new skills or higher levels of responsibility, improving work processes, or other methods.

stakeholders Organizations, groups, or people with a vested interest in the efficiency of the operations or the success of the organization in delivering high-quality patient care.

target population The group of people for whom a training program is intended, usually defined in terms of age, background, and ability. (Also referred to as target audience.)

task   A unit of work activity or operation that forms a significant part of a job function or duty.

training   Instruction and practice for acquiring skills and knowledge of rules, concepts, or attitudes necessary to function effectively in specified task situations.

training content   The knowledge or skill that the trainee must master to be able to meet the training objectives.

training evaluation   The process used to measure the demonstrated ability of individuals and units to accomplish specific training objectives.

training methods   Any of the many instructional approaches or combinations of approaches to achieve learning, such as classroom presentations, technology-based lessons, case study exercises, or self-paced programs.

training objectives   A clearly communicated statement of the desired changes in the target population's skills, knowledge, or abilities. Training objectives often include a description of the *activity* to be demonstrated, the *conditions* under which the activity will be performed, and the *standards* for judging if the activity has been performed at the desired level.

Index

●●●●●●●●●●●●●●●●●●●●●●●●●●●●●●●●●●